BIOLOGICAL ACTIVITIES AND ACTION MECHANISMS OF LICORICE INGREDIENTS

Edited by **Hiroshi Sakagami**

Biological Activities and Action Mechanisms of Licorice Ingredients
http://dx.doi.org/10.5772/64119
Edited by Hiroshi Sakagami

Contributors

Hiroshi Sakagami, Takao Kato, Kunihiko Fukuchi, Taisei Kanamoto, Shigemi Terakubo, Hideki Nakashima, Hirokazu Ohno, Masaji Yamamoto, Yoshinori Nagai, Kiyoshi Takatsu, Yasuharu Watanabe, Hiroe Honda, Tsutomu Hatano, Eerdunbayaer, Yanmei Cui, Teruo Kuroda, Yuuki Shimozu, Ryusuke Oishi, Tetsuji Sato, Noriyuki Kuroda, Yukiyoshi Tamura, Pijush K. Das, Purnima Gupta, Anindita Ukil, Minpei Kuroda, Yoshihiro Mimaki, Yukihiro Shoyama, Hiromitsu Tanaka, Morimasa Wada, Nguyen Huu Tung, Takuhiro Uto, Shunsuke Fujii

Published by InTech
Janeza Trdine 9, 51000 Rijeka, Croatia

Publishing Process Manager Ana Simcic
Technical Editor SPi Global
Cover InTech Design team

First published April, 2017
Printed in Croatia
Legal deposit, Croatia: National and University Library in Zagreb

Additional hard copies can be obtained from orders@intechopen.com

Biological Activities and Action Mechanisms of Licorice Ingredients, Edited by Hiroshi Sakagami
p. cm.
Print ISBN 978-953-51-3119-9
Online ISBN 978-953-51-3120-5

For EU product safety concerns:
IN TECH d.o.o., Prolaz Marije Krucifikse Kozulić 3, 51000 Rijeka, Croatia,
info@intechopen.com or visit our website at intechopen.com.

Meet the editor

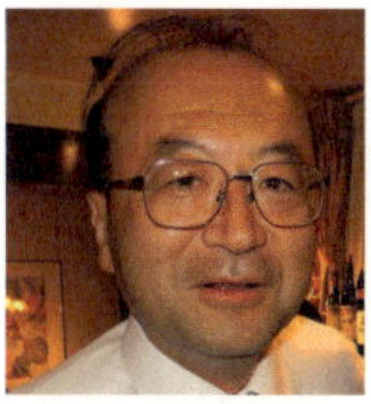

Hiroshi Sakagami received his PhD degree from the Faculty of Pharmaceutical Sciences, University of Tokyo (1980). He worked for 17 years in the Department of Biochemistry, School of Medicine, Showa University, Tokyo, with a 3-year postdoctoral stay in the laboratory of Dr. Aaron Alexander-Bloch, RPMI, Buffalo, NY. He became a professor of Pharmacology, Meikai University School of Dentistry (1997). He is also the chair of MPL research center and director of the board of trustees (Meikai University and Asahi University). His research interest includes the biological function of lignin-carbohydrate complex, application of plant extracts to oral diseases, exploration of anticancer drugs that have least cytotoxicity against normal oral keratinocyte, and creation of new field of research by collaboration with investigators having different backgrounds.

Contents

Preface

Glycyrrhiza is a genus of approximately 18 perennial plant species of the legume family (Fabaceae), mostly grown in Asia, Australia, Europe, and the Americas. The genus is best known for liquorice (British English; licorice in American English). Licorice root extract is used as a single medicine or an additive to as many as 26 Kampo medicines to alleviate pain, allergy, and inflammation. Glycyrrhizin, a major component, is used as a sweetener and taste-masking agent. With rapid progress in the analytical methodology, the action mechanisms of licorice extracts are being elucidated. This book *Biological Activities and Action Mechanisms of Licorice Ingredient* has ten original chapters that are divided into three sections. Section 1 collects three introductory chapters: "Licorice as Alternative Medicine" (Chapter 1), "Its Industrial Application" (Chapter 2), and "Future Market and Trading Prospects of Licorice Between Japan and China" (Chapter 3). Section 2 collects the original review articles of "Structural-Activity Relationship of Licorice Phenolics Focusing on the Antioxidant and Antimicrobial Activity" (Chapter 4), PPAR-γ Ligand-Binding Activity" (Chapter 5), "Antitumor and Antiviral Activity" (Chapter 6), and In Vitro Fertilization Activity" (Chapter 7). Section 3 proposes the action mechanism of immunomodulation induced by licorice components: "Antiadipose Tissue Inflammation and Antifibrosis Activity" (Chapter 8), "Antihepatitis Activity" (Chapter 9), and "Antileishmanial Activity" (Chapter 10).

All of these chapters are written by experts in the multidisciplinary field spanning from the natural sciences to economics and will surely give new insight into licorice and its ingredients to students, clinicians, teachers, and researchers who have interest in alternative medicine.

Hiroshi Sakagami
Division of Pharmacology and Meikai Pharmaco-Medical Laboratory (MPL)
Meikai University School of Dentistry,
Japan

Section 1

History and Future Prospects of Licorice

Chapter 1

Introductory Chapter: Future Prospect of Licorice, Popular Crude Drug and Food Sweetener

Hiroshi Sakagami

Additional information is available at the end of the chapter

http://dx.doi.org/10.5772/67003

1. Classification of drugs

Drugs are classified into "over-the-counter (OTC) drugs" that are sold in drug stores and "medicinal (or ethical) drugs" that are prescribed by doctors [1] (**Figure 1**). "Herbal drug materials" and "Kampo (Japanese Traditional Medicines)" belong to OTC drugs, whereas new drugs and generics belong to the medicinal drugs. In contrast to Western medicines that recognize the drug as single compounds, Kampo medicines are a mixture of more than two components of herbal extracts. Pharmacopeia 17th edition accommodates a total of 323 herbal medicines (33 Kampo medicine + 290 herbal drug materials/formulations). Licorice is a crude drug prescribed in various herbal formulas in traditional Japanese and Chinese medicines and also used worldwide as a food natural sweetener. The origin

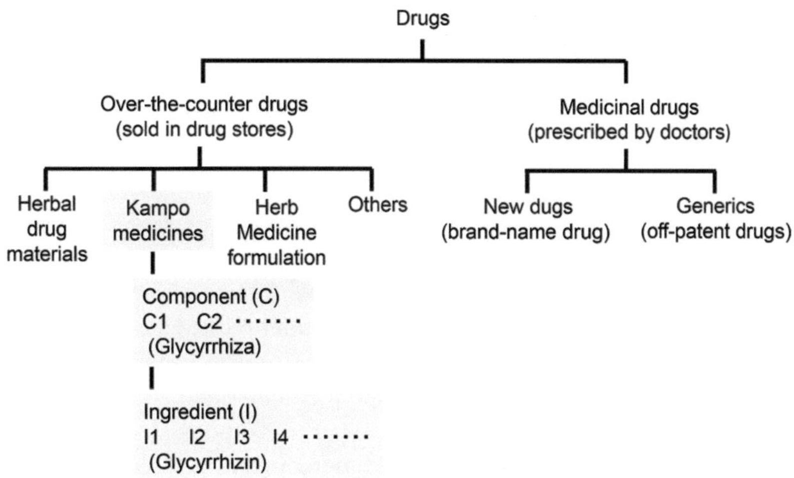

Figure 1. Classification of drugs.

of licorice was the root or stolon of Glycyrrhiza uralensis or G. glabra (Legminosae) [1]. Licorice contains three orders higher amounts of glycyrrhizin, as compared with other components [2].

2. Difference of Kampo medicine and Western medicine

To select the best Kampo medicine, the patient's condition will be first checked by the criteria of yin-yang and xu-shi categorization (activity and physical fitness) and then narrowed down by the life force, blood and colorless bodily fluids, (if necessary) followed by the five viscera theory and the pulse, tongue and belly (**Figure 2**). As compared with Western medicine, Kampo medicine is more empirical (rather than scientific), comprehensive (rather than analytical), global (rather than local) and personal (rather than general) and normalizes the patient's condition (rather than removing the cause of disease).

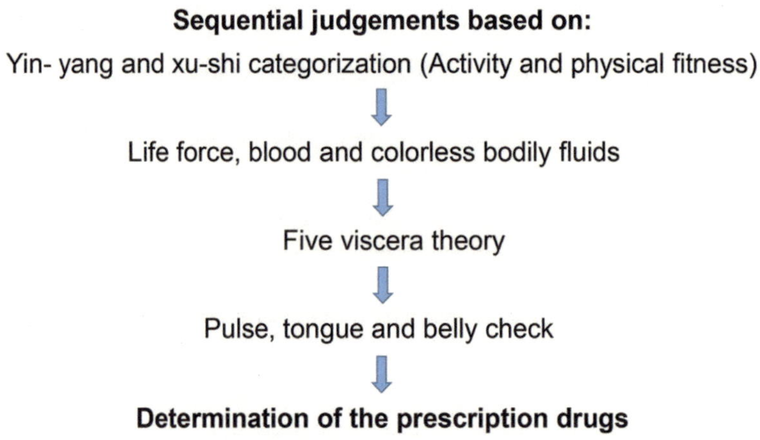

Figure 2. Process of grasping the patient's condition prior to the prescriptions of drugs.

During the business sorting work in 2009, the then Japanese regime proposed the exemption of insurance against Kampo medicines, fomentations and mouth washes, claiming that Kampo medicine is evidence less and it can be obtained very easily by anybody. However, the patients, herbalists and medical personnel moved against this proposal by means of collecting approximately one million signatures and made the proposal withdrawn. Now, in Japan, approximately 150 Kampo medicines and 200 herbal drugs used as decoctions are covered by health insurance. Among the 900 physicians who worked in the core cancer treatment hospitals, 92.4% reported having prescribed Kampo medications [3]. Nationwide, random-sampled and population-weighted telephone survey demonstrated that respondents who had used at least one complementary and alternative medicine (CAM) therapy (76.0%) were greater than those who had used orthodox Western medicine (65.6%) and that the expenditure for CAM was nearly half that of orthodox Western medicine [4]. The most common CAM practice was Kampo, which corresponded to 96.1%

of CAM-practicing doctors [5]. However, it still remains to be clarified why the Kampo medicines exert beneficial effects on our body.

3. Application of Kampo medicines

Kampo medicines have been used to improve the symptoms of various diseases (**Table 1**). Bakumondoto, Hochuekkito and Kiyoshihaiyu, which contains licorice, have been reported to improve the symptoms of chronic obstructive pulmonary disease (COPD) [6, 7]. Daikenchuto (that contains hydroxy-α-sanshool and 6-shogaol as major ingredients) improved the intestinal motor paralysis and Crohn's disease, by increasing the RAMP (receptor activity-modifying membrane protein) 1, 2, 3, mobilizing the CGRP (calcitonin gene-related peptide) and AMD (adrenomedullin) and inhibiting the expression of pro-inflammatory cytokines (TNF-α, IFN-γ) [8]. Rikkunshito recovered the meal uptake by increasing the plasma des-acyl ghrelin level, suggesting its possible application to dyspepsia [9].

Old people experience the decline of body strength and vital function, the continuous languor, the loss of appetite and the fatigability. This kind of aging-associated characteristics cannot be remedied by Western medicines, but more easily alleviated by treating with co-agents such as

	Used to treat or improve the symptom of:	**Presence of Licorice**
Bakumondoto	Chronic obstructive pulmonary disease (COPD)	■
Bofutsushosan	Insulin resistance, obesity	■
Daikenchuto	Increase in intestinal blood flow, Crohn's disease	
Goreisan	Migraine	
Hachimijiogan	Arteriosclerosis, dysuria, prostatomegaly	
Hangekobokuto	Depression	
Hochuekkito	COPD, depression	■
Juzentaihoto	Hepatic fibrosis, carcinogenesis	■
Kakkonto	Migraine	■
Keishibukuryogan	Oxidant stress, vascular endothelial damage in patient arthritis, acne	
Kiyoshihaiyu	COPD	■
Maoto	Inhibition of neuraminidase	■
Rikkunshito	Functional-dyspepsia, gastroesophageal reflux disease, depression	■
Saikokaryukotsuboreito	Depression	
Shosaikoto	Hepatic fibrosis, carcinogenesis	■
Shoseiryuto	Allergic rhinitis	■
Tokishigyakukashokyoto	Sensitivity to cold, numbness	■
Yokukansan	Dementia	■

Table 1. Application of Kampo medicines to various diseases.

Hochuekkito and Juzentaihoto. However, licorice present therein may induce hypokalemia (hypertension, edema, feeling of weakness, convulsions paralysis of the extremities, arrhythmia) [10]. Shosaikoto, which also contains licorice, is known to induce interstitial pneumonia (fever, dry cough, exertional dyspnea) [11]. The use of herbal medicines is increasing all over the world and when a patient with such risk factors is prescribed an herbal medicine containing licorice, careful follow-up is required. The patient's symptoms should be carefully monitored and if no improvement in symptoms is observed, continuous treatment should be avoided.

4. Application to oral diseases

Oral cares are important to maintain the normal oral functions and prevent oral diseases. Recent report suggests an association between oral health and the risk of lacunar infarction [12]. Tooth-blushing and myofunctional therapy stimulate the secretion of saliva [13, 14]. Mouthrinsing with aqueous biocompatible 2-methacryloyloxyethyl phosphorylcholine (MPC)-polymer inhibited the increase in oral bacterial numbers, especially of *S. mutans* [15]. The inhibition of bacterial adherence and biofilm development may prevent the aspiration pneumonia and the periodontitis [16].

However, if the extent of oral diseases exceeds the capacity of oral care, we have to rely on medicines. Various Kampo medicines are used to treat oral diseases such as stomatitis, xerostomia, taste disturbance, halitosis, glossodynia, temporomandibular joint and muscle disorders (TMJ), tooth extraction and periodontal disease (**Table 2**).

	Stomatitis	Xerostomia	Taste disturbance	Halitosis	Glossodynia	TMJ	Tooth extraction	Periodontal disease	Presence of Licorice
Bakumondoto	●	●			●				■
Byakkokaninjinto	●	●	●		●				■
Daisaikoto								●	
Goreisan	●	●			●		●		
Hachimijiogan		●							
Hangekobokuto		●	●	●	●	●			
Hangeshoshinto	●		●	●	●				■
Hochuekkito	●	●			●			●	■
Inchinkoto	●								
Jiinkokato		●							■
Jumihaidokuto	●								■

	Stomatitis	Xerostomia	Taste disturbance	Halitosis	Glossodynia	TMJ	Tooth extraction	Periodontal disease	Presence of Licorice
Juzentaihoto	●	●	●		●				■
Kakkonto	●					●			■
Kamishoyosan	●	●		●	●	●			■
Kanbakutaisoto						●			■
Keishikajutsubuto	●	●			●	●			■
Keishibukuryogan						●			■
Kikyoto							●		■
Kososan	●								■
Orengedokuto	●		●	●				●	
Orento	●			●				●	■
Rikkosan	●				●		●		■
Rikkunshito	●	●	●	●	●				■
Saibokuto			●		●	●			■
Saikokaryukotsuboreito		●	●		●				
Saikokeishikankyoto			●						■
Saikokeishito							●		■
Saireito	●	●							■
Seishinrenshiin		●							■
Shakuyakukanzoto						●			■
Shosaikoto	●		●		●		●		■
Sokeikakketsuto						●			■
Tokishakuyakusan					●	●			
Unseiin	●							●	

Table 2. Application of Kampo medicines to oral diseases.

Hangeshashashashinto showed anti-inflammatory [17], oral ulcer-induced pain-releasing [18], antimicrobial [19], antimucositis [20] and antioxidative activities [21]. Orento prevented the inflammatory responses in lipopolysaccharide-treated human gingival fibroblasts [22]. Rikkosan also induced anti-inflammatory activity [17]. Shosaikoto showed anti-inflammatory [23] and anti-hyperlipidemic and anti-atherosclerotic activities [24]. It should be noted that all these four Kampo medicines contain licorice **(Table 2).**

Kampo medicines are also effective to alleviate the glossodynia [25] and cancer thermotherapy-induced side effects [26–28].

5. Future direction

We sometimes experience that purification of active ingredients leads to significant loss of the biological activity. Furthermore, the amount of ingredients is different from one batch to another depending on where they are harvested. Therefore, it is essential to reconstruct the best sets of active ingredients for the standardization of the contents. First step to accomplish this is to investigate the relationship between the biological activity of structurally related compounds and chemical descriptors, using quantitative structure-activity relationship (QSAR) analysis. Once the best 3D structure is predicted, such compounds should be quickly synthesized to confirm its biological activity. This process is repeated until the satisfactory results are obtained. The next step is to determine the best combination of ingredients (**Figure 3**).

The relative potency of ingredients may depend on the type of target cells. For example, licorice flavonoids showed potent anti-HSV activity, while they were inactive against HIV infection [29]. During isolation of active ingredients, some aggregations between ingredients may happen [30]. Accumulation and analysis of such data are crucial to manufacture the best Kampo medicine.

Using QASR analysis, we recently found that anti-HSV activity of 19 flavonoids including 10 licorice flavonoids correlated well with six chemical descriptors that represent polarizability

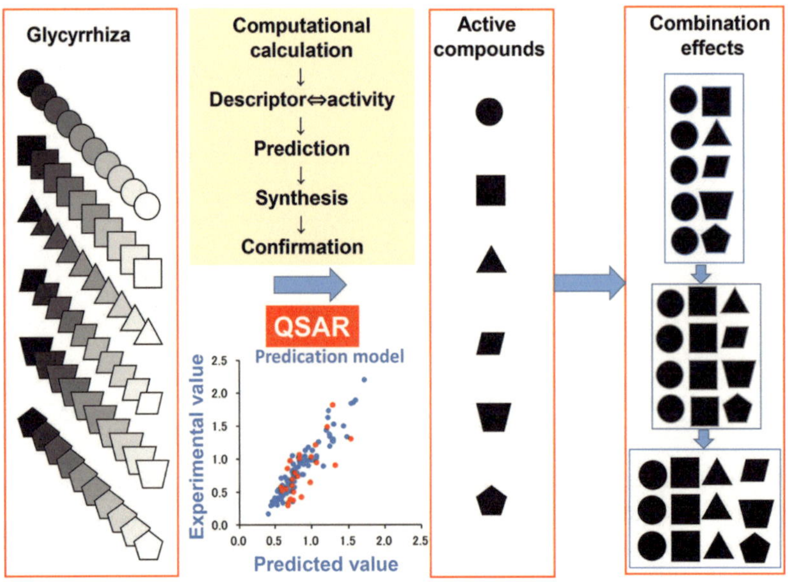

Figure 3. Chart flow to select the best combination of licorice ingredients. Each symbol is any compound. The same shapes indicated the compounds with similar structure.

(MATS5p, GATS5p), ionization potential (GATS5i), number of ring systems (NRS), atomic number (J_Dz(Z)) and mass (J_Dz(m) ($p < 0.0001$). This result suggests that the physico-chemical properties, rather than the category of compound, are important factors in determining the anti-HSV activity [29]. The possibility that their target site may be common is under investigation.

It is expected that in the future, alternative therapy with Kampo medicines will be versioned up, in synchronization with the improvement in the personalized medicine based on the gene information.

Author details

Hiroshi Sakagami

Address all correspondence to: sakagami@dent.meikai.ac.jp

Division of Pharmacology and Meikai Pharmaco-Medical Laboratory (MPL), Meikai University School of Dentistry, Sakado, Saitama, Japan

References

[1] Society of Japanese Pharmacopoeia. The Japanese Pharmacopoeia Sixteenth Edition (JP XVII), Yakuji-Nippo, Tokyo (2016 March).

[2] Kato T, Horie N, Matsuta T, Umemura N, Shimoyama T, Kaneko T, Kanamoto T, Terakubo S, Nakashima H, Kusama K, Sakagami H. Anti-UV/HIV activity of Kampo medicines and constituent plant extracts. In Vivo. 2012;26:1007–1013. PMID: 23160685.

[3] Ito A, Munakata K, Imazu Y, Watanabe K. First nationwide attitude survey of Japanese physicians on the use of traditional Japanese medicine (kampo) in cancer treatment. Evid Based Complement Alternat Med. 2012;2012:957082. doi:10.1155/2012/957082. PMID: 23304230.

[4] Yamashita H, Tsukayama H, Sugishita C. Popularity of complementary and alternative medicine in Japan: a telephone survey. Complement Ther Med. 2002;10(2):84–93. PMID: 12481956.

[5] Watanabe S, Imanishi J, Satoh M, Ozasa K. Unique place of Kampo (Japanese traditional medicine) in complementary and alternative medicine: a survey of doctors belonging to the regional medical association in Japan. Tohoku J Exp Med. 2001;194(1):55–63. PMID: 11556734.

[6] Mukaida K, Hattori N, Kondo K, Morita N, Murakami I, Haruta Y, Yokoyama A, Kohno N. A pilot study of the multiherb Kampo medicine bakumondoto for cough in patients with chronic obstructive pulmonary disease. Phytomedicine. 2011;18(8–9):625–629. doi:10.1016/j.phymed.2010.11.006. Epub 2010 Dec 21. PMID: 21177084.

[7] Tatsumi K, Shinozuka N, Nakayama K, Sekiya N, Kuriyama T, Fukuchi Y. Hochuekkito improves systemic inflammation and nutritional status in elderly patients with chronic obstructive pulmonary disease. J Am Geriatr Soc. 2009;57(1):169–170. doi:10.1111/j.1532-5415.2009.02034.x. PMID: 19170793.

[8] Kono T, Omiya Y, Hira Y, Kaneko A, Chiba S, Suzuki T, Noguchi M, Watanabe T. Daikenchuto (TU-100) ameliorates colon microvascular dysfunction via endogenous adrenomedullin in Crohn's disease rat model. J Gastroenterol. 2011;46(10):1187–1196. doi:10.1007/s00535-011-0438-2. PMID: 21808981.

[9] Togawa K, Matsuzaki J, Kobayakawa M, Fukushima Y, Suzaki F, Kasugai K, Nishizawa T, Naito Y, Hayakawa T, Kamiya T, Andoh T, Yoshida H, Tokura Y, Nagata H, Mori M, Kato K, Hosoda H, Takebayashi T, Miura S, Uemura N, Joh T, Hibi T, Suzuki H. Association of baseline plasma des-acyl ghrelin level with the response to rikkunshito in patients with functional dyspepsia. J Gastroenterol Hepatol. 2016;31(2):334–341. doi:10.1111/jgh.13074. PMID: 26252950.

[10] Ottenbacher R, Blehm J. An unusual case of licorice-induced hypertensive crisis. S D Med. 2015;68(8):346–347, 349. PMID: 26380428.

[11] Nakayama M, Bando M, Hosono T, Yamasawa H, Ohno S, Sugiyama Y. Evaluation of the drug lymphocyte stimulation test (DLST) with shosaikoto [in Japanese]. Arerugi. 2007;56(11):1384–1389.

[12] Taguchi A, Miki M, Muto A, Kubokawa K, Migita K, Higashi Y, Yoshinari N. Association between oral health and the risk of lacunar infarction in Japanese adults. Gerontology. 2013;59(6):499–506. doi:10.1159/000353707. PMID: 23942139.

[13] Inenaga K, Inangaki T, Hosokawa R, Ono K. Parotid salivary secretion induced by stimulation of periodontal regions with toothbrush in humans. J Med Invest. 2009;56(Suppl):277. PMID: 20224201.

[14] Carnaby-Mann G, Crary MA, Schmalfuss I, Amdur R. "Pharyngocise": randomized controlled trial of preventative exercises to maintain muscle structure and swallowing function during head-and-neck chemoradiotherapy. Int J Radiat Oncol Biol Phys. 2012;83(1):210–219. doi:10.1016/j.ijrobp.2011.06.1954. PMID: 22014959.

[15] Hirota K, Yumoto H, Miyamoto K, Yamamoto N, Murakami K, Hoshino Y, Matsuo T, Miyake Y. MPC-polymer reduces adherence and biofilm formation by oral bacteria. J Dent Res. 2011;90(7):900–5. doi:10.1177/0022034511402996. PMID: 21447697.

[16] Martínez JA, Soto S, Fabrega A, Almela M, Mensa J, Soriano A, Marco F, Jimenez de Anta MT, Jordi V. Relationship of phylogenetic background, biofilm production and time to detection of growth in blood culture vials with clinical variables and prognosis associated with Escherichia coli bacteremia. J Clin Microbiol. 2006;44(4):1468–1474. doi:10.1128/JCM.44.4.1468-1474.2006, PMCID: PMC1448679.

[17] Kato T, Segami N, Sakagami H. Anti-inflammatory Activity of Hangeshashinto in IL-1β-stimulated Gingival and Periodontal Ligament Fibroblasts. In Vivo. 2016;30(3):257–263. PMID: 27107084.

[18] Hitomi S, Ono K, Yamaguchi K, Terawaki K, Imai R, Kubota K, Omiya Y, Hattori T, Kase Y, Inenaga K. The traditional Japanese medicine hangeshashinto alleviates oral ulcer-induced pain in a rat model. Arch Oral Biol. 2016;66:30–7. doi:10.1016/j.archoralbio.2016.02.002. PMID: 26878477.

[19] Fukamachi H, Matsumoto C, Omiya Y, Arimoto T, Morisaki H, Kataoka H, Kadena M, Funatsu T, Fukutake M, Kase Y, Kuwata H. Effects of hangeshashinto on growth of oral microorganisms. Evid Based Complement Alternat Med. 2015;512947. doi:10.1155/2015/512947. PMID: 26170876.

[20] Matsuda C, Munemoto Y, Mishima H, Nagata N, Oshiro M, Kataoka M, Sakamoto J, Aoyama T, Morita S, Kono T. Double-blind, placebo-controlled, randomized phase II study of TJ-14 (Hangeshashinto) for infusional fluorinated-pyrimidine-based colorectal cancer chemotherapy-induced oral mucositis. Cancer Chemother Pharmacol. 2015;76(1):97–103. doi:10.1007/s00280-015-2767-y. PMID: 25983022.

[21] Matsumoto C, Sekine-Suzuki E, Nyui M, Ueno M, Nakanishi I, Omiya Y, Fukutake M, Kase Y, Matsumoto K. Analysis of the antioxidative function of the radioprotective Japanese traditional (Kampo) medicine, hangeshashinto, in an aqueous phase. J Radiat Res. 2015;56(4):669–77. doi:10.1093/jrr/rrv023. PMID: 25883171.

[22] Ara T, Honjo K, Fujinami Y, Hattori T, Imamura Y, Wang PL. Preventive effects of a kampo medicine, orento on inflammatory responses in lipopolysaccharide treated human gingival fibroblasts. Biol Pharm Bull. 2010;33(4):611–616.

[23] Ara T, Maeda Y, Fujinami Y, Imamura Y, Hattori T, Wang PL. Preventive effects of a Kampo medicine, Shosaikoto, on inflammatory responses in LPS-treated human gingival fibroblasts. Biol Pharm Bull. 2008;31(6):1141–4. PMID: 18520044.

[24] Shen YR, Inoue M, Nagatsu Y, Ogihara Y, Aburada M. Anti-hyperlipidemic and anti-atherosclerotic actions of shosaikoto (kampo medicine). Biol Pharm Bull. 1996;19(9):1160–1165. PMID: 8889034.

[25] Hijikata Y, Makiura N, Kano T, Higasa K, Shimizu M, Kawata K, Mine T. Kampo medicine, based on traditional medicine theory, in treating uncured glossodynia: efficacy in five clinical cases. Am J Chin Med. 2008;36(5):835–847.

[26] Ohnishi S, Takeda H. Herbal medicines for the treatment of cancer chemotherapy-induced side effects. Front Pharmacol. 2015 Feb;10;6:14. doi:10.3389/fphar.2015.00014. PMID: 25713534.

[27] Aoyama T, Nishikawa K, Takiguchi N, Tanabe K, Imano M, Fukushima R, Sakamoto J, Oba MS, Morita S, Kono T, Tsuburaya A. Double-blind, placebo-controlled, randomized phase II study of TJ-14 (hangeshashinto) for gastric cancer chemotherapy-induced oral mucositis. Cancer Chemother Pharmacol. 2014;73(5):1047–1054. doi:10.1007/s00280-014-2440-x. PMID: 24652604.

[28] Kono T, Takeda H, Uezono Y. Kampo medicine for the treatment of adverse effects caused by anticancer drugs [in Japanese]. Nihon Geka Gakkai Zasshi. 2013;114(5):251–255. PMID: 24167978.

[29] Fukuchi K, Okudaira N, Adachi K, Odai-Ide R, Watanabe S, Ohno H, Yamamoto M, Kanamoto T, Terakubo S, Nakashima H, Uesawa Y, Kagaya H, Sakagami H. Antiviral and antitumor activity of licorice root extracts. In Vivo. 2016;30:777–786.

[30] Sakagami H, Zhou Li, Kawano M, Thet MM, Takana S, Machino M, Amano S, Kuroshita R, Watanabe S, Chu Q, Wang QT, Kanamoto T, Terakubo S, Nakashima H, Sekine K, Shirataki Y, Hao ZC, Uesawa Y, Mohri K, Kitajima M, Oizumi H, Oizumi T. Multiple biological complex of alkaline extract of the leaves of Sasa senanensis Rehder. In Vivo 2010;24:735–744.

Chapter 2

The History of Licorice Applications in Maruzen Pharmaceuticals Co., Ltd.

Yukiyoshi Tamura

Additional information is available at the end of the chapter

http://dx.doi.org/10.5772/65962

Abstract

Licorice is the root and stolon of the genus *Glycyrrhiza* plants. Licorice has a long and storied history of use in both Eastern and Western cultures for over 4000 years. Licorice extracts and its principal component, glycyrrhizin, have been used extensively in foods, tobacco, and cosmetics and in both traditional and herbal medicines. Since its start-up in 1938, our company has been working on extracting and purifying the flavoring, sweetening, cosmetic, and medicinal constituents from licorice. At first, we were manufacturing licorice extracts for soy sauce. Recently, our company has developed new licorice products, such as antioxidative and antimicrobial products for foods from hydrophobic licorice extracts; whitening, antioxidative, and antityrosinase products for cosmetics from hydrophobic licorice extracts; antiaging products for cosmetics from licorice leaves; and some disease-suppression products for agriculture and fishery by water-soluble licorice flavonoids. This chapter presents the history of several kinds of food and cosmetic applications from many extracts and purified constituents from licorice plants in our company.

Keywords: *Glycyrrhiza* plants, glycyrrhizin, flavonoids, application, foods, cosmetic

1. Introduction

Licorice (liquorice in British English, Gancao in Chinese, the leguminous plant (Fabaceae)) is a perennial plant grown in the Mediterranean region, the Middle East, Central Asia, Russia, and China. Licorice is the root and stolon of the genus *Glycyrrhiza* plants. Licorice has a long and storied history of use in both Eastern and Western cultures for over 4000 years. Licorice extracts and its principle component, glycyrrhizin, have been used for extensive use in foods, tobacco, and cosmetics and in both traditional and herbal medicines [1–3]. As for the components of *Glycyrrhiza* species, about 100 kinds of triterpenoid saponins and sapogenins and about 300 kinds of phenolic compounds have been reported [4]. Since its start-up in 1938, our company has been working on extracting and purifying the flavoring, sweetening, cosmetic and medicinal constituents from licorice. In the early days, the licorice extracts have been used in the food industry, which includes soy sauce and salted foods. Also the licorice extracts and glycyrrhizin have been used in the cosmetic industry. Recently, our company has developed new licorice products, such as antioxidative and antimicrobial products for foods from hydrophobic licorice extracts; whitening, antioxidative and antityrosinase products for cosmetics from hydrophobic licorice extracts; antiaging products for cosmetics from licorice leaves; and some-disease suppression products for agriculture and fishery by water-soluble licorice flavonoids. Our company is a world-leading company to supply a high quality of licorice products and has a historical know-how of licorice-derived product manufacturing (**Figure 1**). This chapter presents the history of several kinds of food and cosmetic applications from many extracts and purified constituents from licorice plants in our company.

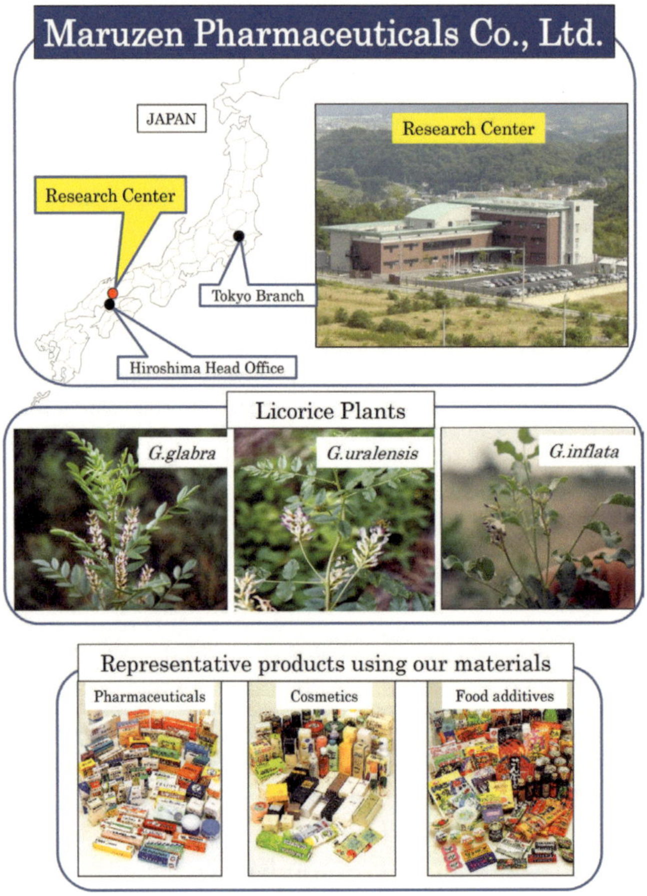

Figure 1. Maruzen Pharmaceuticals profile, licorice plants, and its formulated finished products.

http://dx.doi.org/10.5772/65962

2. Glycyrrhizin-producing *Glycyrrhiza* plants

Licorice is applied to the root and stolon of some *Glycyrrhiza* species. Among around 30 species of genus *Glycyrrhiza* [5], the three species of genus *Glycyrrhiza* are commercially used, because they contain glycyrrhizin, which is the main sweetening and bioactive agent. The water-soluble constituents of the three *Glycyrrhiza* species, *G. uralensis, G. glabra,* and *G. inflata* are almost same. On the other hand, the hydrophobic extract from the three *Glycyrrhiza* species contains the species-specific flavonoids (**Table 1**) [6]. The structures of these compounds are shown in **Figure 2**. Glycyrrhizin is a conjugate of two molecules, glucuronic acid and glycyrrhetic acid, an oleanane-type triterpene. Glycyrrhizin is found in the thickening root and the stolon, but not in the seed, leaf, and stem. Hydrophobic flavonoids are found in the peel of the root and stolon.

***Glycyrrhiza* plant**	**Distribution**	**Water soluble constituents**		**Hydrophobic flavonoids**
		Saponin	**Flavonoids**	
G. uralensis	China, Mongolia, Kazakhstan	Glycyrrhizin	Liquiritigein and its glycosides isoliquiritigenin and its glycosides	Glycycoumarin licocoumarone
G. glabra	Mediterranean region Middle East Central Asia	Glycyrrhizin	Liquiritigein and its glycosides isoliquiritigenin and its glycosides	Glabridin glabrene
G. inflata	Xinjiang(China)	Glycyrrhizin	Liquiritigein and its glycosides isoliquiritigenin and its glycosides	Licochalcone A licochalcone B

Table 1. Distribution and constituents of the three kinds of *Glycyrrhiza* species.

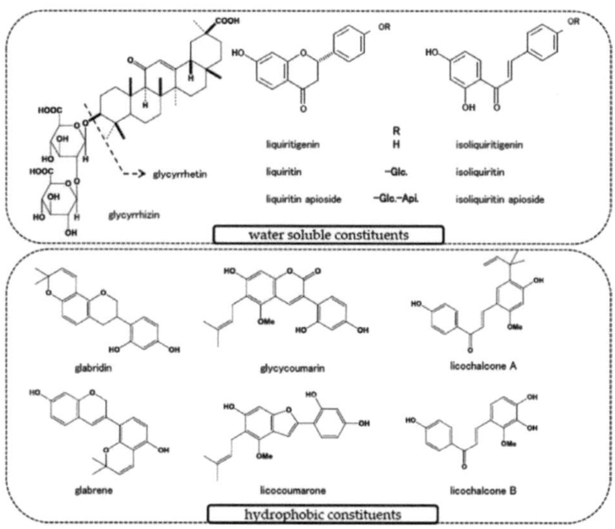

Figure 2. Structures of the constituents of the three kinds of *Glycyrrhiza* species.

3. Application of licorice products for foods

Pontefract cakes are made of licorice extract, molasses, sugar, and flour in the Yorkshire town of Pontefract, England, during the seventeenth century. In the nineteenth century, it was used extensively for confectionery [7]. Licorice extracts and glycyrrhizin have the following properties [8]:

1. High-intensity sweetener, glycyrrhizin possesses about 200 times the sweetness potency of sucrose
2. Improving foam stabilization and head-forming characteristics
3. Masking effect of bitter aftertaste
4. Flavor-enhancing effect
5. Nonfermented sweetener
6. Noncaramelization
7. Heat stable
8. Soften the saltiness
9. Depression of freezing point
10. Full-bodied umami and sweetening

Therefore, licorice extracts and glycyrrhizin are used as food additives in a variety of foods such as alcohol beverages, nonalcohol beverages, chewing gum, candy, chocolate, sweet snacks, ice cream, soy sauce, Japanese pickled vegetables, seafood delicacies, steamed fish paste, and sausages in Japan.

Research work by our company in 1994 resulted in a yeast that selectively hydrolyzed the terminal β-glucuronyl linkage of glycyrrhizin to yield glycyrrhetic acid 3-*O*-mono-glucuronide (MGGR), a potent sweetener (relative sweetness to sucrose: ×950, **Table 2**) [9, 10]. Moreover, MGGR has a flavor-enhancing property (**Table 3**) [11].

Comparable sucrose concentration (%)	In water		In 5% salt solution	
	Glycyrrhizin	MGGR	Glycyrrhizin	MGGR
2	250	1400	–	–
4	170	950	500	2800
6	170	950	500	2800
8	150	730	440	2400
10	100	500	320	1400

Table 2. Relative sweetness intensity in water or 5% salt solution.

	Cocoa	Chocolate	Whipped cream
Blank	2*	2*	16**
MGGR	7*	8*	27**
Same	1*	0*	17**

*No. of panelist felt delicious.
**Delicious score.

Table 3. Flavor-enhancing effect of MGGR against cocoa, chocolate, and whipped cream.

4. Application of licorice products for pharmaceuticals and cosmetics

Glycyrrhizin has also demonstrated antiviral, antimicrobial, anti-inflammatory, antiallergy, antiulcer, antitussive, hepatoprotective, and blood pressure-increasing effects *in vitro* and *in vivo*. In addition, glycyrrhizin is effective in treating hyperlipidemia and inflammation-induced skin hyperpigmentation and is effective in preventing neurodegenerative disorders and dental caries [2].

Therefore, licorice extract, glycyrrhizin, and its derivatives are extensively used in the preparation of cosmetics in Japan. Glycyrrhizin as well as licorice extracts, glycyrrhetin, stearyl glycyrrhetinate, and succinyloxy -glycyrrhetinate (carbenoxolone) are used in drugs, quasi-drugs, and cosmetics. Glycyrrhizin and its salts are used in eye drops, lotions, and tonics as they are soluble in water. On the other hand, glycyrrhetic acid and its derivatives are used in creams, milky lotions, and sun oils as they are soluble in oil.

5. Application of hydrophobic extract of licorice for cosmetics and foods

Recently, the species-specific flavonoids from hydrophobic extracts of *G. uralensis, G. glabra*, and *G. inflata* were found. The primary active ingredient isolated from *G. uralensis* was glycycoumarin, that isolated from *G. glabra* was glabridin, and that isolated from *G. inflata* was licochalcone A (**Figure 1**). In the course of our studies on the further application of licorice as a cosmetic ingredient, we studied new dermatological availabilities in the hydrophobic extracts of licorice containing licochalcone A isolated from *G. inflata* and glabridin isolated from *G. glabra*.

5.1. Efficacies of hydrophobic extract from *G. inflata* (HPGI)

The primary active ingredient isolated and extracted from *G. inflata* is licochalcone A, an oxygenated retrochalcone that exhibits antimicrobial, antioxidative, anti-inflammatory, antiparasitic activity, and antitumorigenic activity [12, 13].

We indicate several efficacies of hydrophobic extracts from *G. inflata* (HPGI), especially in dermatological uses. The efficacy of HPGI against sebum-induced skin trouble was assessed in several experiments (**Table 4**) [14]. An androgenic hormone, testosterone, is converted into a pharmacologically active compound, dihydrotestosterone, by an intracellular enzyme, testosterone 5α-reductase. Dihydrotestosterone combines with the androgen receptor of the sebaceous gland to increase the sebum. Ultimately, the increase of sebum-secretion promotes skin trouble through the oxidative damage and increase of acne fungus.

Tests	**Inhibitory effect (IC_{50}: ppm)**
Testosterone 5α-reductase activity	18.7
Androgen receptor	5.8
Lipase activity	43.6
Phospholipase A activity	0.38
SOD-like activity	7.0
Antimicrobial activity against *P. acnes*	15.6 (MIC)

Table 4. Inhibitory effects of HPGI on sebum-induced skin trouble experiments.

(1) Inhibitory test of testosterone 5α-reductase. As shown in **Table 4**, in an assay of the inhibitory effect against testosterone 5α-reductase activity, HPGI demonstrated the potent inhibitory activity. The inhibitory ability was more effective than positive controls (ethynyl estradiol (IC_{50}: 31.5 ppm) and benzyl peroxide (IC_{50}: 129 ppm)).

(2) Inhibitory effect against androgen receptor.

In this assay, HPGI inhibited the binding of dihydrotestosterone on the receptor at a low concentration and its IC_{50} was 5.8 ppm (**Table 4**). From this result, it was indicated that HPGI has a binding ability in the androgen receptor and works an androgen antagonist.

(3) Inhibitory effect against lipase and phospholipase A_2.

HPGI indicated the inhibition of lipase (IC_{50}: 43.6 ppm) and phospholipase A_2 (IC_{50}: 0.38 ppm). In this case, the potency of HPGI against phospholipase A_2 was remarkable.

(4) Superoxide dismutase (SOD) like activity.

The suppressant effect of HPGI on active oxygen generation was examined by the reduction of nitro blue tetrazolium (NBT) in a xanthine-xanthine oxidase system. In this assay, HPGI suppressed the generation of active oxygen at low concentration (IC_{50}: 7.0 ppm).

(5) Antimicrobial activity against *Propionibacterium acnes*.

In the hair follicle and the sebaceous gland, *P. acnes* produces the chemotactic factor that enhances the migration of neutrophils toward the hair follicle or the sebaceous gland, and causes the development of acne. In addition, *P. acnes* is considered to increase the release of cytokine and T-lymphocyte. These cells and the sebaceous gland also promote damage by acne through allergic reaction. Furthermore, *P. acnes* can multiply in the hair follicle by using the sebum as a nutriment and enhance the production of enzyme, such as lipase, protease, and hyaluronidase. Among these enzymes, lipase attacks sebum to give free fatty acid and promotes the formation of the primary eruption, comedo. Besides, free radicals generated from fatty acid attack phospholipid in cell membranes result in the formation of chemical mediators, such as prostaglandins and leukotrienes. These mediators derived by the action of phospholipase A_2 enhance the development of acne through inflammatory reaction.

HPGI has antimicrobial activity against *P. acnes* at a low concentration (MIC: 31.3 ppm).

(6) Efficacy assessment in acne patient.

From the above-mentioned results *in vitro* assays, HPGI expected following four actions: (1) inhibitory action of sebum production, (2) antimicrobial action, (3) inhibitory action of allergic and inflammatory response, and (4) suppressant action of oxidative damage.

Therefore, we assessed the efficacy of HPGI in acne patients.

Twenty female acne patients received anti-acne gel containing HPGI. All patients applied anti-acne gel onto the whole face twice or three times daily for 2 weeks.

Table 5 shows the result of efficacy assessment in acne patients. In 17 of the 20 patients tested, the improvement effect was recognized [13].

Efficacy	No. of patients
Marked improvement	6
Improvement	5
Slightly improvement	6
No effect	3
Worse	0

Table 5. Result of efficacy assessment of HPGI preparation in acne patients (n = 20).

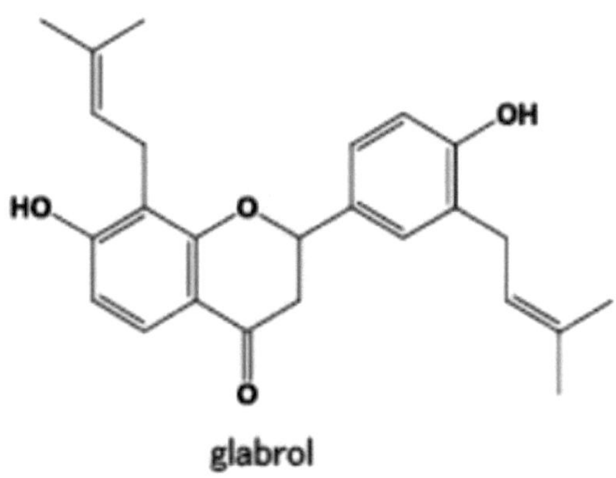

Figure 3. Structure of flavonoid in HPGG.

5.2. Efficacies of hydrophobic extracts from *G. glabra* (HPGG)

The hydrophobic extract from *G. glabra* (HPGG) contains various flavonoids such as glabridin, glabrene, and glabrol (**Figure 3**). HPGG has been known to have antimicrobial and antioxidant activities [15]. In addition, glabridin has the inhibitory effects on melanogenensis and inflammation [16]. In this section, a depigmenting effect of HPGG *in vitro* and *in vivo* studies was examined [17].

(1) Inhibitory effect of tyrosinase activity.

We found that HPGG and its constituents had inhibitory effects on tyrosinase activity by absorbance measurement. Their tyrosinase inhibition doses (IC_{50}: mg/mL) were as follows: glabridin 0.0003, HPGG 0.031, glabrene 0.0046, hydroquinone 0.016, and ascorbic acid 0.21 (**Table 6**) [15]. The latter two compounds are commonly known as depigmenting agents.

Sample	IC_{50} (mg/mL)
HPGG	0.0031
Glabridin	0.0003
Glabrene	0.0046
Glabrol	>0.1
Ascorbic acid	0.21
Kojic acid	0.058
Hydroquinone	0.016

Table 6. Inhibition against tyrosinase activity.

(2) Melanization assay by 14C-thiouracil uptake.

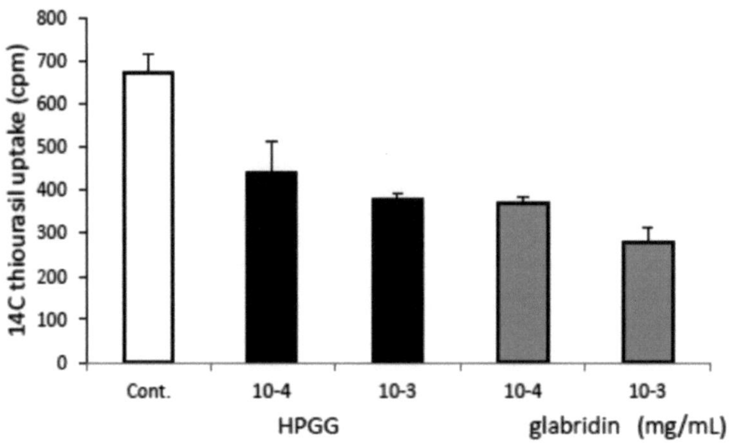

Figure 4. Melanization assayed by ^{14}C-thiouracil uptake of B-16 melanoma cells.

http://dx.doi.org/10.5772/65962

Melanization was assayed by the incorporation of ^{14}C-thiouracil into B-16 melanoma cells. Melanization was inhibited by HPGG and glabridin dose-dependently, although glabridin more strongly inhibited it than HPGG (**Figure 4**) [15].

(3) Application in patients with melasma.

We have first synthesized an HPGG that contains 40% of glabridin and using this HPGG, 0.1 or 0.2% HPGG creams were made. An open study has been carried out with application of 0.1 or 0.2% HPGG cream twice a day in patients with melasma, senile pigment freckle, and postinflammatory pigmented lesions for 4 months. The efficacy was evaluated by measuring skin lightness (*L* value) with colorimeter before and after the application. The *L* value has a theoretical value ranging from of 0 (pure black) to 100 (pure white).

L value was significantly improved after the therapy with 0.1% HPGG cream in patients with melasma only (**Table 7**) [15]. However, with 0.2% HPGG cream, not only patients with melasma, but also with the two lesions showed significantly improvement in *L* values (**Table 8**) [15].

Disease	No. of cases	*L* value before and after the 4 month therapy
Chloasma	20	Before 58.28 ± 4.06 $p < 0.05$
		After 59.25 ± 3.61
Postinflammatory pigmentation	6	Before 57.56 ± 3.44 NS
		After 58.22 ± 2.46
Chloasma + PIP	7	Before 60.26 ± 2.09 NS
		After 60.62 ± 3.44
Total	33	Before 58.57 ± 3.65 $p < 0.05$
		After 59.35 ± 3.39

Table 7. Changes in *L* values by application with 0.1% GPGG cream.

Disease	No. of case	*L* value before and after the 4 month therapy
Chloasma	12	Before 55.80 ± 3.09 $p < 0.01$
		After 57.37 ± 2.68
Postinflammatory pigmentation	8	Before 56.34 ± 3.84 $p < 0.05$
		After 57.94 ± 3.06
Senile pigment freckle	15	Before 55.75 ± 3.48 $p < 0.05$
		After 56.99 ± 2.63
Total	35	Before 55.90 ± 3.34 $p < 0.01$
		After 57.33 ± 2.69

Table 8. Changes in *L* values by application with 0.2% GPGG cream.

6. Application of licorice leaf extract for cosmetics

The aerial parts of licorice are less used in cosmetics. A few phytochemical investigations on the *G. glabra* leaves have reported the presence of several phenolic constituents that are not present in the root [18–20].

We found that licorice extract from *G. glabra* has antiaging effect on human skin [21]. Skin hydration is one of the most important claims in cosmetics as hydrated skin gives an impression of healthy skin. Intracellular lipids in stratum corneum (SC), which are composed mainly of cholesterol, fatty acids, and ceramide, play a crucial role for both water-holding and permeability barrier function in SC. Hyaluronan (HA) is also known to have high water-retaining capacity released to skin hydration, elasticity, and plasticity. It has been reported that HA decreased and was found to be changed in aged skin. Therefore, materials that can modulate ceramide and HA contents in SC could be very effective for aging skin.

6.1. Isolation of licorice leaf components

Ten components were isolated from 70% ethanol extract of licorice leaf from *G. glabra*. Three active components out of 10 are shown in **Figure 5** [19].

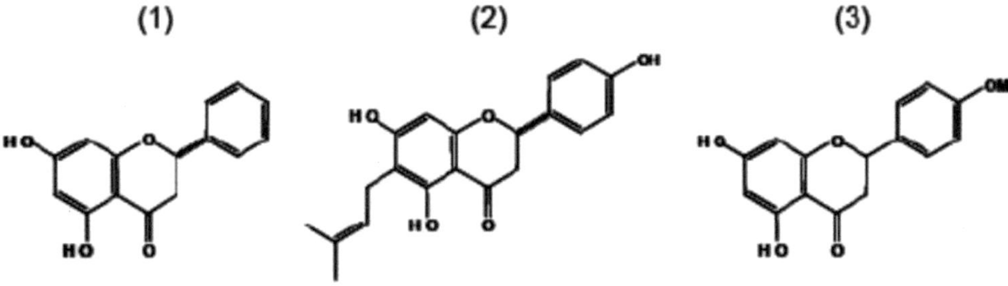

Figure 5. Structure of isolated active components from licorice leaf extract. (1) Pinocembrin, (2) 6-prenyl-naringenin, (3) angophorol.

6.2. Effects of licorice leaf extract on mRNA expressions of ceramide-related enzymes

To examine the effects of plant extracts on ceramide synthesis, real-time quantitative RT-PCR analysis was performed on gene expressions of serine palmitoyltransferase long chain base subunit 1 (SPTLC1) and SPTLC2, which were two subunits of serine palmitoyltransferase (SPT) and acid sphingomyelinase (SMPD1). SPT is known to catalyze the rate-limiting step of de novo ceramideynthesis. Acid sphingomyelinase (SMPD1) is also known to convert sphingomyelin into ceramide and plays an important role in ceramide generation for permeability barrier function. Licorice leaf extract and 6-prenyl-naringenin showed the promoting activity on mRNA expressions of SPTLC1, SPTLC2, and SMPD1 in a dose-dependent manner (**Table 9**) [19].

http://dx.doi.org/10.5772/65962

	mRNA expressions (% of control)			
	Licorice leaf extract (μg/mL)		6-prenyl-naringenin (μg/mL)	
	5	20	2.5	5
SPTLC1	113.3 ± 3.5*	132.9 ± 2.7***	113.7 ± 3.7*	148.4 ± 3.7***
SPTLC2	108.8 ± 3.9	127.6 ±11.6	113.9 ±14.5	93.8 ±12.4
SMPD1	117.3 ± 4.1	132.9 ± 8.1*	153.8 ± 9.4**	353.3 ± 5.9***

*$p < 0.05$
**$p < 0.01$
***$p < 0.001$

Table 9. Effects of licorice leaf extract on the mRNA levels of SPTLC, SPTLC2, and SMPD1.

These results indicate that licorice leaf extract may increase de nove biosynthesis of ceramide and hydrolysis of sphingomyelin to ceramide.

6.3. Effect of licorice leaf extract on ceramide production in skin-equivalent models and human skin

To examine whether licorice leaf extract has an efficacy on the production of ceramide in skin-equivalent models. The extract dramatically promoted the production of ceramide in skin-equivalent models (**Figure 6**) [19]. For further research to determine the efficacy on the production of ceramide in human skin, 1% licorice leaf extract or placebo lotion was topically applied on healthy volunteers (n = 10). The amount of ceramide by the topical application of 1% licorice leaf extract lotion (1.58 μg/mg) was increased as compared to that of placebo lotion (0.56 μg/mg) (**Figure 7**) [19].

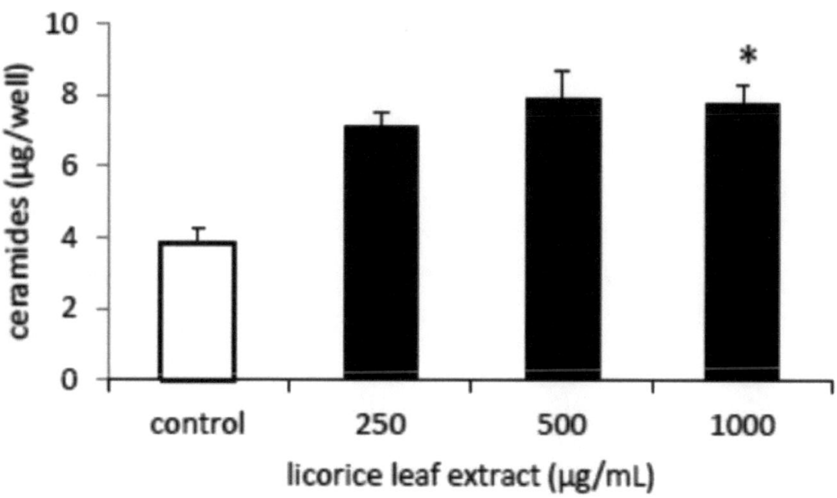

Figure 6. Effects of licorice leaf extract lotion on ceramide production. *$p < 0.05$ compared with the control.

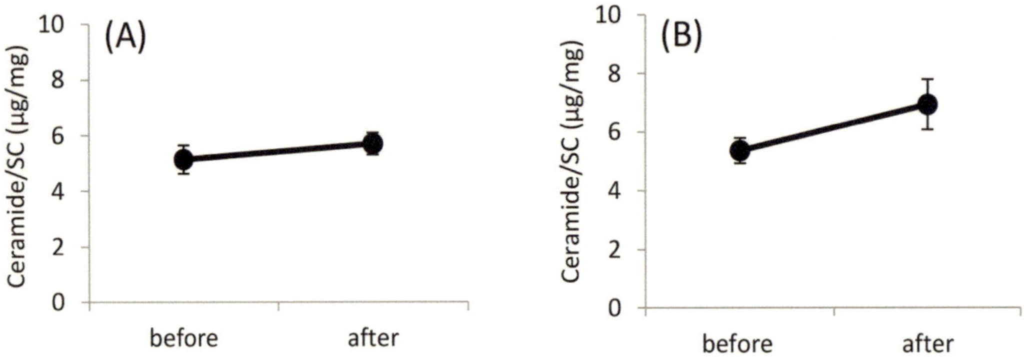

Figure 7. Effects of licorice leaf extract lotion on ceramide production. Placebo lotion (A) and 1% licorice leaf extract lotion (B). Values were the mean SEM; $n = 10$.

These results suggested that licorice leaf extract has an efficacy on the synthesis of ceramide.

6.4. Effects of licorice leaf extract on mRNA expression of 3-hydroxy-3-methylglutaryl-CoA reductase (HMGCR), a key enzyme on cholesterol biosynthesis

To examine whether licorice leaf extract has a promoting effect on other stratum corneum lipids, real-time quantitative RT-PCR analysis was performed on mRNA expression of HMGCR, the key enzyme for de novo cholesterol synthesis. Treatment with licorice leaf extract showed a significant increase in the expression of HMGCR mRNA by 150% compared with the controls (**Figure 8(A)**). Among three components tested, especially 6-prenyl-naringenin enhanced the expression of HMGCR mRNA in the dose-dependent manner (**Figure 8(B)**) [19]. These results indicate that licorice leaf extract and its components may increase biosynthesis of cholesterol as well as ceramide. Further studies will be needed to determine the promoting activity on cholesterol synthesis.

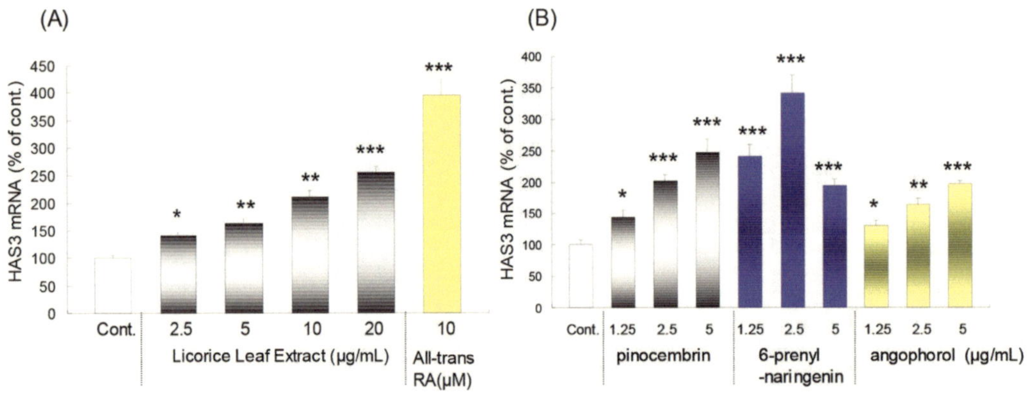

Figure 8. Effects of licorice leaf extract (A) and the components (B) on the mRNA level of HMGCR. *$p < 0.05$; **$p < 0.01$; ***$p < 0.001$, compared with the controls.

6.5. Effects of licorice leaf extract on HA production

Gene expression of HAS3 that relates to hyaluronan biosynthesis was upregulated by the treatment of licorice leaf extract in the dose-dependent manner in normal human epidermal keratinocytes (NHEK) (**Figure 9(A)**). Three components tested also enhanced the hyaluronan synthase 3 (HAS3) mRNA expression (**Figure 9(B)**) [19]. All-trans retinoic acid that is known as a stimulator of HA synthesis in NHEK also showed a strong increase in the expression of HAS3 mRNA by 400% compared with the control. To examine whether licorice leaf extract has a promoting activity on HA production, ELISA analysis was performed using cell culture supernatant. These results indicate that licorice leaf extract and its components have a potent stimulation activity for HA production.

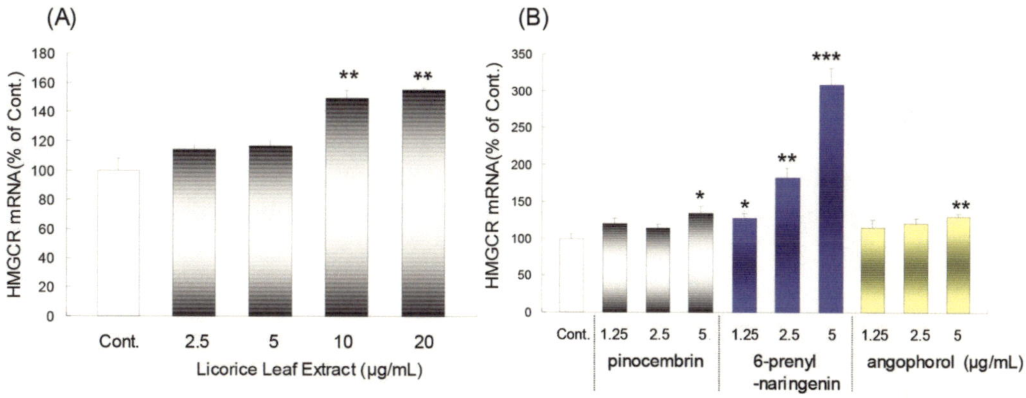

Figure 9. Effects of licorice leaf extract (A) and the components (B) on the mRNA level of HAS3 in NHEK. $*p < 0.05$; $**p < 0.01$; $***p < 0.001$, compared with the control.

These results indicate that licorice leaf extract may be a useful ingredient for skin hydration and barrier repair because of their ability to synthesize ceramide through the enhancement of mRNA expressions of SPT and SMPD1 and the increase of mRNA of HMGCR related to cholesterol biosynthesis and the increase of HA production through the enhancement of mRNA levels of HAS3 by its active principles.

7. Application of flavonoid-rich water-soluble licorice flavonoids (WSLF) for agriculture and fishery

Table 10 shows the flavonoid composition of water-soluble licorice flavonoids (WSLF) tested. WSLF contains about 10% of the total flavonoids and 10% of glycyrrhizin. General water extracts of licorice contain 2% of the total flavonoids and 10% of glycyrrhizin. WSLF tested has five times higher content of total flavonoids [22].

Compounds	Contents (%)
Flavonoids	
Liquiritin	4–8
Isoliquiritin	1–3
Liquiritigenin	0.5–2.0
Isoliquiritigenin	0.5–2.0
Saponin	
Glycyrrhizin	8–13

Table 10. Contents of flavonoids and saponin of water-soluble licorice flavonoids (WSLF).

7.1. Control of some fungal foliage diseases of vegetables using WSLF

7.1.1. In vitro test of WSLF

The antifungal activity *in vitro* of WSLF was evaluated by culture tests using the PDA agar medium. The antifungal activity of WSLF among various pathogens causing fungal foliage diseases on vegetables was investigated. WSLF exhibited the antifungal activity against 15 fungi tested (**Table 11**) [23].

Plants	Diseases	Pathogen	% Inhibition of mycerial growth	
			100 μg/mL	1000 μg/mL
Rice	Blast	*Magnaporthe grisea*	14	61
	Bakanae disease	*Gibberella fujikuroi*	37	84
	Sheath blight	*Thanatephorus cucumeris*	16	71
	Seed and seedling rot	*Pythium graminicola*	16	17
Tomato	Late blight	*Phytothora infestans*	18	55
	Gray mold	*Botrytis cinerea*	18	45
	Corynespora target spot	*Corynespora cassicola*	34	67
	Leaf mold	*Passalora fulva*	29	60
Egg plant	Leaf mold	*Mycovellosiella nattrassii*	19	58
Sweet pepper	Frogeye leaf spot	*Cercospora capsici*	11	42
Cucumber	Corynespora leaf spot	*Corynespora cassicola*	20	51
	Anthracnose	*Colletotrichum orbiculare*	11	71
Melon	Gummy stem blight	*Didymella bryoniae*	50	50
Spinach	Fusarium wilt	*Fusarium oxysporum f. spinaciae*	38	59
Potato	Late blight	*Phytothora infestans*	29	43

Table 11. The antifungal activity of WSLF.

http://dx.doi.org/10.5772/65962

WSLE solution of 20 μL of spore solution and 20 μL was mixed on the slide maintained at 25°C for 20 h. The germinated spores were counted under a microscope. WSLE at 0.1 and 1% inhibited the germination of spores in three kinds of fungi (**Table 12**) [23].

Plants	Diseases	Concentration (%)	Inhibition rate (%)	
			No. 1	No. 2
Sweet pepper	Frogeye leaf spot	0.1	48.4	50.1
		1	87.8	94.2
Water			2.3	5.9
Egg plant	Leaf mold	1	76.2	72.3
Water			2.9	4.4
Cucumber	Corynespora Leaf spot	1	62.4	
Water			26.4	

Table 12. Effect of WSLE on the germination of spores.

7.1.2. Control of fungal foliage diseases in vivo

Control efficacy of WSLE against seven pathogens was evaluated in pot tests. WSLE solutions were sprayed onto young plants. After air-drying the solutions, the plants were artificially inoculated with the spore suspension on the test pathogen, and incubated at 25°C for a given period. Percent of disease control was assessed after the inoculation of 9–12 days by visually measuring the number of diseasing spot.

Control efficacy of WSLE among seven pathogens exhibited 80–100% at 1% (**Table 13**) [24]. In the pot test, WSLE showed excellent control of diseases caused by various pathogens.

Plant disease	No. of disease spot	Inhibition rate (%)
Tomato Corynespora target spot		
WSLE 1%	30	98
Water	1926	
Tomato late blight (no. 1)		
WSLE 1%	0	100
Water	9.3	
Tomato late blight (no. 2)		
WSLE 1%	0	100
Water	22.8	
Cucumber Corynespora leaf spot		
WSLE 1%	506.0	80

Plant disease	No. of disease spot	Inhibition rate (%)
Water	2541.0	
Cucumber anthracnose		
WSLE 1%	4.0	97
Water	134.5	
Cucumber downy mildew		
WSLE 1%	0	100
Water	31.1	
Sweet pepper frogeye leaf spot		
WSLE 1%	17.5	97
Water	520.0	

Table 13. Efficacy of WSLE against 6 pathogens.

7.2. Efficacy of WSLE on fish diseases

7.2.1. Antibacterial activity of WSLE against fish disease causing bacteria in vitro

The antibacterial activity of WSLE was examined by the agar dilution method, which ranged from 32 to 1024 μg/mL against 33 kinds of bacteria. As shown in **Table 14**, WSLE inhibited the growth of Gram-positive bacteria with MIC values of 128–512 μg/mL. Whereas of the Gram-negative bacteria 17 kinds of bacteria were sensitive and nine kinds of bacteria were insensitive to the inhibitory effect [25].

Bacteria	MIC (μg/mL)	Bacteria	MIC (μg/mL)
Gram-positive bacteria			
Carnobacterium pisciicola	256	*Staphylococcus epidermidis*	512
Nocardia asteroides	256	*S. aureus*	256
Bacillus cereus	256	*Lactococcus garvieae*	128
B. brebis	256		
Gram-negative bacteria			
Aeromonas hydrophila	>1024	*Vibrio. damsela*	1024
A. salmonicida	1024	*V. fisheri*	128
Flavobacterium columnare	64	*V. fluviaris*	>1024
F. psychrophilum	64	*V. carchariae*	>1024
Flexibacter maritimus	256	*V. harveyi*	1024
Pseudomonas chloraruphis	>1024	*V. ichthyoenteri*	512
Photobacterium damsela	1024	*V. ordalli*	256

Bacteria	MIC (μg/mL)	Bacteria	MIC (μg/mL)
Enterococcus cloacae	>1024	*V. parahaemolyticus*	1024
Escherichia coli	>1024	*V. penaeicida*	256
Klebsiella planticola	>1024	*V. proteolitycus*	>1024
Salmonella typhimurium	1024	*V. splendidus*	512
Vibrio alginolyticus	>1024	*V. tubiashii*	256
V. anguillarum	1024	*V. vulnificus*	256

Table 14. Antibacterial activity of WSLE.

The MICs of constituents, liquiritigenin, and isoliquiritigenin are shown in **Table 15**. Isoliquiritigen demonstrated significant antibacterial activity against all bacteria tested. In contrast, liquiritigenin exhibited no antibacterial activity against six kinds of bacteria tested [23].

Bacteria	MIC (μg/mL)	
	Liquiritigenin	**Isoliquiritigenin**
Gram-positive bacteria		
Nocardia asteroides	128	<32
Staphylococcus epidermidis	>128	64
S. aureus	>128	128
Gram-negative bacteria		
Aeromonas salmonicida	>128	>128
Photobacterium damsela	>128	128
Vibrio anguillarum	>128	128
V. harveyi	>128	>128

Table 15. Antibacterial activities of constituents in WSLE.

7.2.2. Effects of WSLE on nonspecific immune responses and disease resistance against Edwardsiella tarda infection in Japanese flounder, Paralichthys olivaceus

7.2.2.1. Effects of WSLE on nonspecific immune responses in Japanese flounder, P. olivaceus

Healthy Japanese flounder, each weighting about 56 g, was divided into three groups used in 0, 5, and 50 mg/kgBW/day of WSLE. Each diet was fed to three groups once a day for 2 weeks. After 1 and 2 weeks of feeding, five fishes from each group were randomly collected. Blood was drawn from the caudal vein and used for hemolytic and lysozyme activities. Hemolytic activity of WSLE-treated fish was significantly higher ($P < 0.05$) than that of the control fish after 1 and 2 weeks (**Figure 10**) [24]. On the other hand, lysozyme activity showed little change (**Figure 11**) [24].

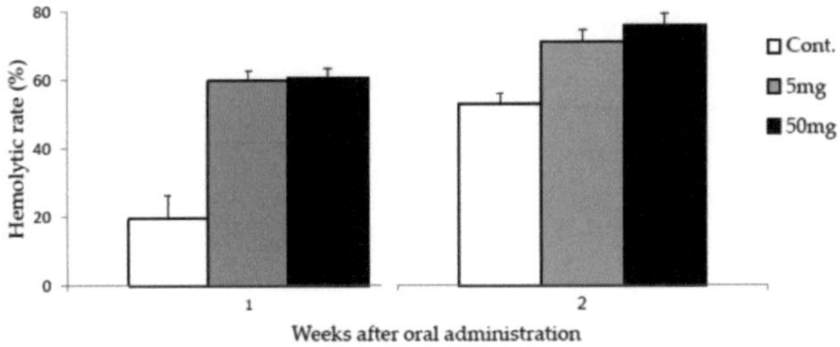

Figure 10. Hemolytic activity of Japanese flounder serum.

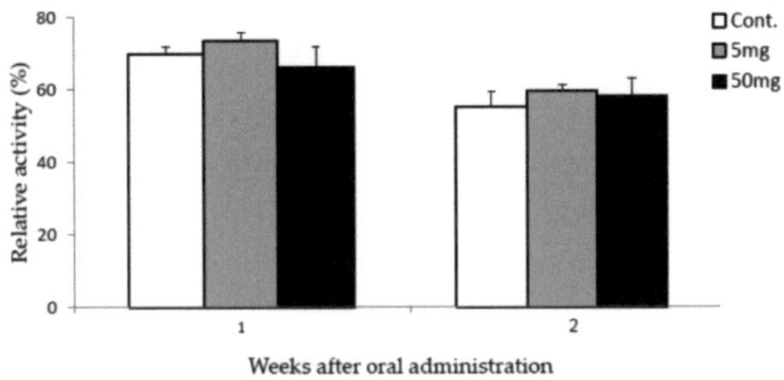

Figure 11. Lysozyme activity of Japanese flounder serum.

Leukocytes were collected from the head kidney and the intestinal tract and used for superoxide anion release and phagocytic activities. The production of the superoxide anion was quantified by the reduction of nitro blue tetrazolium (NBT). WSLE showed significant higher activity than the control group after 1 and 2 weeks (**Figure 12**) [25]. The activity increased according to time in most groups. The production of the superoxide anion is a method for destroying intracellular bacteria. Phagocytic activities of head-kidney and intestinal tract leukocytes were determined under a microscope by the zymosan-NBT method. Supplementation of WSLE significantly ($p < 0.05$) enhanced the phagocytic activity after 1 and 2 weeks (**Figure 13**) [26].

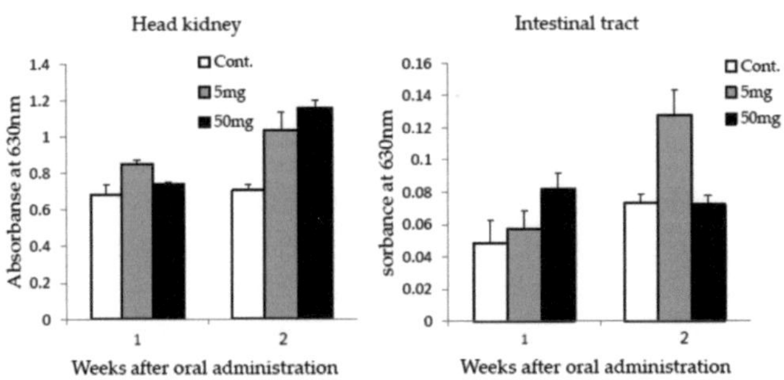

Figure 12. NBT reduction activity of Japanese flounder leukocytes.

http://dx.doi.org/10.5772/65962

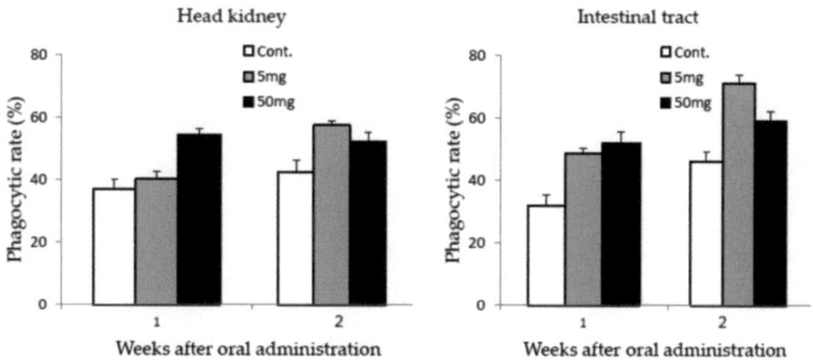

Figure 13. Phagocytic activity of Japanese flounder leukocytes.

7.2.2.2. Effects of WSLE on disease resistance against Edwardsiella tarda infection in Japanese flounder, P. olivaceus

Healthy Japanese flounder, each weighing about 53 g, was divided into three groups of 33 fishes fed with 0, 5, and 10 mg/kgBW/day of WSLE, respectively. These three groups were fed with each supplementation diet once a day for 10 days. On the 10th day of feeding, these groups were injected intraperitoneally with 8.0×10^2 CFU of *E. tarda*.

The cumulative survival rate of the experimental fish following *E. tarda* intraperitoneal challenge is shown in **Figure 14** [27, 28]. The cumulative survival rate was high 48 and 44% when infected fish were fed with 5 and 10 mg/kgBW/day diet and low as 20% in 0 mg/kgBW/day diet fed group, respectively.

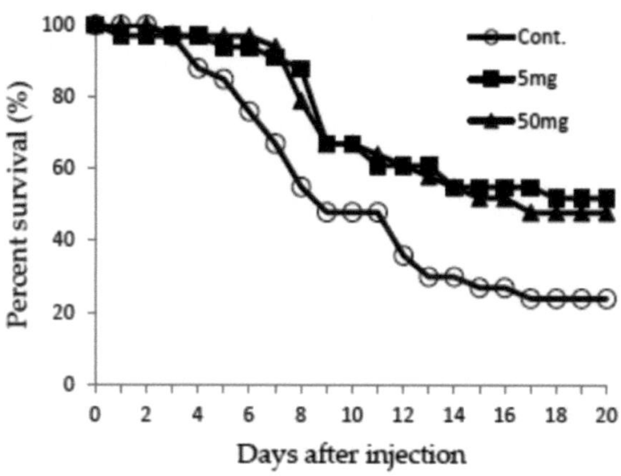

Figure 14. Effect of WSLE administration on the survival of Japanese flounder experimentally infected with *E. tarda*.

Oral administration of WSLE caused enhancement in humoral (hemolytic and lysozyme) and cellular (phagocytic and superoxide anion release) activities. After 10 days of dietary treatment with WSLE, the fish were challenged by intraperitoneal injection with *E. tarda*, WSLE-treated fish demonstrated increased survival rate.

8. Conclusion

Licorice has been used for pharmaceuticals, cosmetics, and food products as water-soluble licorice extract that contains glycyrrhizin, the primary constituent having sweet-taste and various biological activities. Recently, many studies have focused on the licorice ingredients except glycyrrhizin, about 300 phenolic compounds were found from licorice. We investigated licochalcone A extracted from *G. inflata* and glabridin from *G. glabra* in particular. The primary active ingredient isolated and extracted from *G. inflata* is licochalcone A, an oxygenated retrochalcone, which has been associated with various biological properties such as an antioxidant, antimicrobial, as well as anti-inflammatory. As a result, licochalcone A showed several activities such as inhibitory effects of testosterone 5α-reductase, lipase, and phospholipase A_2, as well as androgen receptor antagonist, antimicrobial and SOD-like activities, which relate to skin care, especially the suppression of acne formation and development. On the basis of this evidence, a trial of licochalcone A with acne patients was carried out and the efficacy was demonstrated clinically. The primary active ingredient of *G. glabra* is glabridin, a prenylated isoflavonoid, which is one of the most studies licorice flavonoids, a comprehensive literature survey linked to its bioactivities. Glabridin has inhibitory effects on tyrosinase activity, a key enzyme in the production of melanins and melanization using cultured B16 melanoma cells. An open study of glabridin with melasma patients was conducted. The efficacy was evaluated by measuring skin lightness before and after therapy. Glabridin significantly improved after the therapy not only in melasma but also in lesions. The aerial parts of licorice have received scant interest. The few phytochemical investigations on the *G. glabra* leaves have shown the presence some flavonoids that are not in the roots. We found licorice leaf extract and its component, 6-prenyl-naringenin upregulated both SPTLC1 and SMPD1 mRNA expression related to ceramide synthesis as well as HMGCR mRNA expression related to the cholesterol synthesis. In addition, licorice leaf extract stimulated ceramide production in skin-equivalent models and human skin and promoted HA synthesis by a mechanism that involves upregulation of HAS3 mRNA expression. These results suggested that the licorice leaf extract may be a useful ingredient for skin hydration and barrier repair. There are few reports on licorice extract and glycyrrhizin used in agriculture and fishery. We examined flavonoid-rich water soluble licorice extract (WSLE) in agriculture and fishery uses. In agriculture, WSLE suppressed hyphal elongation of 12 kinds of plant pathogenic fungi and zoospore release from the conidia. In the pot test, WSLE suppressed the number of lesions in six kinds of plant diseases. As a result, we suggested WSLE has the control effects on some fungal diseases of vegetables such as cucumber, tomato, and sweet pepper. In fishery, WSLE and isoliquiritigenin inhibited the fish disease caused by bacteria, especially Gram-positive bacteria. Effects of WSLE on nonspecific immune response of Japanese flounder were investigated. Oral administration of 5 or 50 mg/kgBW/day of WSLE for 2 weeks showed some significant enhance in humoral (hemolytic and lysozyme activities) and cellular (super oxide anion release and phagocytic activities) activities. After 10 days dietary treatment with WSLE, the fishes were challenged by intraperitoneal injection with *E. tarda*, WSLE-treated fish demonstrated increased survival rate.

http://dx.doi.org/10.5772/65962

9. Future direction

As for licorice resources, licorice plants are widely found growing wild in regions along the Silk Road. However, according to the recent overharvesting of wild licorice, its habitants are severely disturbed and many of them are degraded or undergoing desertification, especially in China. Therefore, licorice cultivation has been undertaken in China. However, in the present glycyrrhizin and flavonoid content of the cultivated licorice is lower than wild one. In the aim of securing a stable source of licorice, we have to study to obtain the cultivated licorice with same quality of wild licorice.

Over the past half-century, we have been engaged in the development of licorice extracts and its components, and have been offering a number of useful and unique materials to our customers in medicinal, cosmetic, functionary food, and food industries. Elucidation of the constituents and biological activities of both underground and aerial parts in licorice plants have led to the development of many valuable licorice products for various industries. We are further expanding the potential of licorice.

Author details

Yukiyoshi Tamura

Address all correspondence to: y-tamura@maruzenpcy.co.jp

Research Center, Maruzen Pharmaceuticals Co., Ltd., Fukuyama, Hiroshima, Japan

References

[1] Shibata S. A Drug over the Millennia: Pharmacognosy, Chemistry and Pharmacology of Licorice. Yakugaku Zasshi. 2000;120:849–862.

[2] Isbrucker RA, Burdock GA. Risk and Safety Assessment on the Consumption of Licorice Root (*Glycyrrhiza* sp.), Its Extract and Powder as a Food Ingredient, with Emphasis on Pharmacology and Toxicology of Glycyrrhizin. Regulatory Toxicology and Pharmacology. 2006;46:167–192.

[3] Hayashi H, Sudo H. Economic Importance of Licorice. Plant Biotechnology. 2009;26:101–104.

[4] Nomura T, Fukai T. Phenolic Constituents of Licorice (*Glycyrrhiza* species), In: Herz W, Kirby GW, Moore RE, Steglich W, Tamm Ch (eds.), Progress in the Chemistry of Organic Natural Products 73. Springer Wien, New York; 1998. pp. 1–140.

[5] Satake M. Glycyrrhiza Plants. In: Records of Lecture in 2nd Meeting on Crude Drug; December 6; Tokyo. 1986. pp. 1–21.

[6] Tamura Y. New Developments in Licorice. Bokin Bobai. 2005;33:127–136.

[7] Nieman C. Licorice. Advances in Food Research. 1959;7:339–381.

[8] Fenwick GR, Lutomski J, Nieman C. Licorice, *Glycyrrhiza glabra* L.—Composition, Uses and Analysis. Food Chemistry. 1990;38:119–143.

[9] Kuramoto T, Ito Y, Oda M, Tamura Y, Kitahata S. Microbial Production of Glycyrrhetic Acid 3-*O*-Mono-β-D-Glucuronide from Glycyrrhizin by *Cryptococcus Magnus* MG-27. Bioscience, Biotechnology and Biochemistry. 1994;58:455–458.

[10] Mizutanii K, Kuramoto T, Tamura Y, Ohtake N, Doi S, Nakaura M, Tanaka O. Sweetness of Glycyrrhetic Acid 3-*O*-β-Monoglucuronide and the Related Glycosides. Bioscience, Biotechnology and Biochemistry. 1994;58:554–555.

[11] In-house Data. Application of Glycyrrhizin and Stevioside in Foods. 1994; pp.1–12.

[12] Tsukiyama R, Katsura H, Tokuriki N, Kobayashi M. Antibacterial Activity of Licochalcone A Against Spore-Forming Bacteria. Antimicrobial Agents and Chemotherapy. 2002;46:1226–1230.

[13] Baumann LS. Less-Known Botanical Cosmeceuticals. Dermatologic Therapy. 2007;20:330–342.

[14] Kambara T, Zhou YY, Kawashima Y, Kishida N, Mizutani K, Ikeda T, Kameyama K. A New Dermatological Availability of the Flavonoids from Licorice Roots-Effect on Acne. Journal of Society Cosmetic Chemists Japan. 2003;37:179–186.

[15] Okada K, Tamura Y, Yamamoto M, Inoue Y, Takagaki R, Takahashi K, Demizu S, Kajiyama K, Hiraga Y, Kinoshita T. Identification of Antimicrobial and Antioxidant Constituents from Licorice of Russian and Xinjiang Origin. Chemical and Pharmaceutical Bulletin. 1989;37:2528–2530.

[16] Yokota T, Nishio H, Kubota Y, Mizoguchi M. The Inhibitory Effect of Glabridin from Licorice Extracts on Melanogenesis and Inflammation. Pigment Cell Research. 1998;11:355–361.

[17] Haramoto I. Licorice Extract has an Inhibitory Effect on Melanogenesis and Improves Melasma Other Pigmented Lesions by Its Topical Use. The St. Marianna Medical Journal. 1994;22:941–948.

[18] Fukui H, Goto K, Tabata M. Two Antimicrobial Flavanones from the Leaves of *Glycyrrhiza glabra*. Chemical and Pharmacological Bulletin. 1998;36:4174–4176.

[19] Biondi DM, Rocco C, Ruberto G. New Dihydrostilbene Derivatives from the Leaves of *Glycyrrhiza glabra* and Evaluation of Their Antioxidant Activity. Journal of Natural Products. 2003;66:477–480.

[20] Siracusa L, Saija A, Cristani M, Cimino F, D'Arrigo M, Trombetta D, Rao F, Ruberto G. Phytocomplexes from Liquorice (*Glycyrrhiza glabra* L.) Leaves—Chemical Characterization and Evaluation of Their Antioxidant, Anti-genotoxic and Anti-inflammatory Activity. Fitoterapia. 2011;82:546–556.

[21] Kiso A, Kawashima Y, Ohto N, Zhou YY, Tohi K, Murakami T, Araho D, Kambara T, Mizutani K. The Effects of Licorice Leaf Extract on Ceramide and Hyaluronan Synthesis. Journal of Society Cosmetic Chemists Japan. 2009;43:267–273.

[22] Miyagawa H. Control of Foliage Diseases of Vegetables by Using a New Licorice Extract, Licorice Extract MZ-1. Food Research. 2009;653:36–39.

[23] Miyagawa H, Ohno H. Control of Some Fungal Foliage Diseases of Vegetables Using Purified Licorice Extract. Bulletin of the National Agricultural Research Center for Western Region. 2007;6:55–69.

[24] Miyagawa H, Ohno H. Studies on the Mechanism of Cucumber Downy Mildew and Anthracnose Suppression by Licorice Extract. Bulletin of NARO Western Region Agricultural Research Center. 2014;13:71–106.

[25] Furushita M, Maeda T, Shiba T, Ohno H, Yamamoto M, Tamura Y. Antimicrobial Activity of a New Licorice Extract-Flavolicorice. Gekkan Aqua Culture. 2005;42:76–77.

[26] Miyoshi Y, Fukuda Y, Ohno H, Kawahara E, Kusuda R. Effect of Oral Administration of Licorice Extract on Non-Specific Immune Response of Japanese Flounder, *Paralichthys olivaceus*. In: Annual Meeting of the Japanese Society of Fish Pathology; September; Nagasaki. 2006.

[27] Miyoshi Y, Kawahara E, Fukuda Y. Effect of Oral Administration of Licorice Extract on the Non-Specific Immunodefense Activity of Japanese Flounder, *Paralichthys olivaceus*. Oita Fisheries Experimental Station Research Report. 2009;1–4.

[28] Miyoshi Y, Ohno. Effect of a New Licorice Extract on Disease Resistance in Marine Fishes. Aqua Culture. 2010;47:57–59.

Chapter 3

Trading of Licorice between Japan and China: Future Market Prospects

Ryusuke Oishi

Additional information is available at the end of the chapter

http://dx.doi.org/10.5772/66514

Abstract

Recent years have seen changes in the trade of licorice between Japan and China. Particularly, the price of imported Chinese licorice has been increasing every year. As the price of Chinese licorice is expected to remain high, Japanese importers may find it increasingly difficult to import licorice from China, leading to a decline in the use of Chinese licorice in Japan. Instead of focusing on the pharmacological properties of licorice, we examine data such as the price and trading volume between China and Japan in order to analyze the licorice market from an economic perspective. From our analysis, we conclude that the recent increase in the price of Chinese licorice in Japan is mainly due to the combined effect of an increase in demand and a decrease in the supply of the product. We demonstrate the need for a cultivated strain as a substitute for native Chinese strains to ensure the continued supply of licorice in Japan.

Keywords: licorice, trade, supply, demand, cultivation, economics

1. Introduction

Licorice has been used as a medicine for over 2000 years. The first mention of its use as a drug for treating wounds is found in a Chinese traditional medicine book from the second century BC [1]. Similarly, licorice has been widely used in Japan, including in the pharmaceutical industry [2]. Despite the high demand, there is no strain of licorice that is native to Japan, meaning that the licorice used in Japanese pharmaceutical products is mostly imported from places such as China and the Middle East [2]. However, recent years have brought changes to the market, as excessive harvesting has depleted the licorice resources in China [3]. This has caused the price of licorice to increase year by year. As the price of Chinese licorice is expected to remain high, it will become difficult for the Japanese pharmaceutical industry to continue to purchase Chinese licorice. In the worst case, the supply of Chinese licorice will be severely constrained.

To avoid this situation, consumers of Chinese licorice in Japan must seek an alternative source. However, this is not an easy task since other countries are hardly able to supply a substitute for Chinese licorice. This study focuses, instead, on attempts to cultivate licorice as a means to mitigate the high price of Chinese licorice.

In this paper, we examine data, such as the price and trading volume of licorice between China and Japan, to analyze the licorice market from an economic perspective. While numerous publications have analyzed the various properties of licorice, studies incorporating economic ideas are rare. To make this study understandable to readers who are unfamiliar with economics, we attempt to limit ourselves to basic economic concepts rather than more specialized ones.

The rest of this paper is organized as follows. In Section 2, we consider the recent situation surrounding Japanese licorice imports from China by examining relevant trade data. In Section 3, we briefly explain some basic economic ideas, which are then discussed in Section 4. Section 5 considers potential solutions, such as efforts to cultivate licorice, and Section 6 concludes the chapter.

2. Changes in the trading volume of licorice between Japan and other countries

Licorice is used in the manufacture of various pharmaceutical products and is indispensable for pharmaceutical industries in many countries, including Japan [2]. There is no variety of licorice that is indigenous to Japan [2]. Licorice used in the manufacture of pharmaceutical products is usually found in the grasslands and sandy soils of southern Europe, Central Asia, and China [4].

Because of this, Japanese pharmaceutical firms have had to rely on imports from abroad [2].

Table 1 shows the cumulative total amount of licorice imported into Japan, in tons, from its 12 major trading partners in the period 2007–2015.[1]

Among the trading partners listed in **Table 1**, China is by far the largest exporter. This indicates that Japan is highly dependent on China for its supply of licorice.

A closer investigation of **Table 1** also reveals that among the listed trading partners, only China and Afghanistan continuously exported licorice to Japan during this period. China's large and continuous supply of licorice played an important role in the Japanese market.

On examining other data from **Table 1** (i.e., Japan's licorice imports from countries other than China), we find that a large proportion of imports is from Central Asian countries, such as

[1] **Table 1** is derived from Trade Statistics of Japan conducted by the Japanese Ministry of Finance (http://www.customs.go.jp/toukei/srch/index.htm?M=01&P=0) [Accessed: 2016-09-17].

Afghanistan, Uzbekistan, and Turkmenistan. This is likely due to these countries' agricultural suitability for licorice (i.e., native strains of licorice grow well in sandy soils) [4]. However, closer examination reveals that the supply of licorice from these countries is not stable but varies from year to year. In addition, the amount of licorice supplied by these countries is much smaller than that supplied by China.

Countries	2007	2008	2009	2010	2011	2012	2013	2014	2015
Azerbaijan					17.85	2		10	
Afghanistan	300	495	396.57	288.84	199.9	104.04	311.57	100	210
Uzbekistan			21.5		22.2	99	10		8.1
Australia	144.71	48.52	7.47						
Kazakhstan			20			21.25			
South Korea								0.08	
China	932.5	1,138.38	868.95	1,239.26	1,770.6	2,181.58	1,936.88	1,547.86	1,397.55
Turkmenistan			100	100	517.5				
Pakistan			8		100	216	45.53	15	
Myanmar		0.04							
Mongolia			3.3			0.23			
Russia				3.87	30.55		0.02	0.2	37.47

Table 1. Cumulative Total Amount of Licorice Imported to Japan, in tons,from its Major Trading Partners (2007–2015).

In addition to the listed Asian and Middle Eastern countries, Australia and Russia also export licorice to Japan. Australia and Russia are attractive trading partners for Japan since these countries are large, with abundant natural resources. However, the sharp fluctuations of trading volume seen in **Table 1** indicate that stable trading between those countries and Japan remains difficult.

As demonstrated above, China is Japan's most important trading partner for licorice.

This is not only due to China's large and stable supply of licorice but also because of its geographical advantage, that is, China is closer to Japan than other suppliers, thus reducing the time and cost of transportation.

However, there is a point of concern in the licorice trade between Japan and China. Particularly, on examining the data in **Table 1**, we find that the volume of Japanese imports of licorice from China peaked in 2012. This is likely an indication of a decrease in the supply of licorice in China.

From 2007 to 2015, Japanese imports of Chinese licorice far exceeded imports from Asia and the Mideast.

Figure 1A and **B** shows the proportions of Japanese imports of licorice from the exporters in 2007 and 2015, respectively. The latter figures incorporate data from **Table 1**.

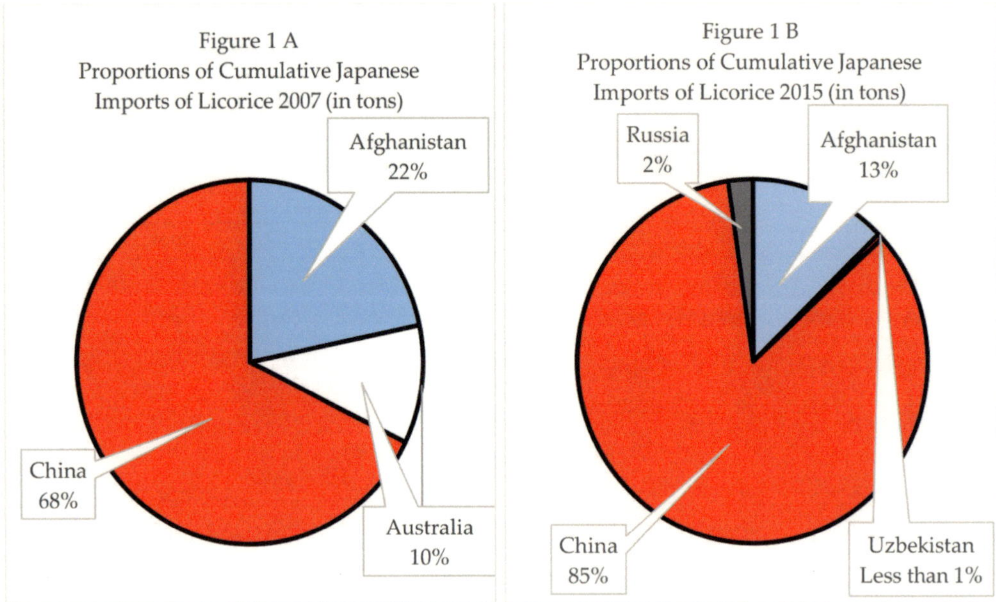

Figure 1. (A) Proportions of cumulative Japanese imports of licorice 2007 (in tons). (B) Proportions of cumulative Japanese imports of licorice 2015 (in tons).

Figure 1A and **B** reveals that Japan strongly relies on China to procure licorice. In addition, comparison of the latter figures also reveals that a proportion of Japanese licorice import from China increases from 2007 to 2015. In other words, in the period between 2007 and 2015, Japanese reliance of China to procure licorice became stronger.

To understand the current trading situation of licorice between Japan and other countries, we can also look at the total amount of money spent importing licorice. **Table 2** shows the cumulative total value (in 1000 yen) for the data presented in **Table 1**.[2]

As seen in **Table 2**, the cumulative total value of Japanese licorice imports from China is much greater than that from other countries and reflects the large trade volume with China.

In addition, we also provide **Figure 2A** and **B** which shows the proportions of Japan's cumulative total spending for importing licorice from the trading partners in relation to the data presented in **Table 2** in 2007 and 2015, respectively.

As can be seen from **Figure 2A** and **B**, in both 2007 and 2015, Japan's cumulative total spending for importing licorice is mostly for the one from China. However, as compared from the proportions in **Figure 1A** and **B**, the proportions of cumulative total spending for importing licorice from China in **Figure 2A** and **B** are larger. The latter indicates that, as compared from other trading partners, such as Afghanistan, Australia, Russia, and Uzbekistan, the price of licorice from China is relatively higher.

[2] **Table 2** is derived from Trade Statistics of Japan conducted by the Japanese Ministry of Finance (http://www.customs.go.jp/toukei/srch/index.htm?M=01&P=0) [Accessed: 2016-09-17].

http://dx.doi.org/10.5772/66514

Countries	2007	2008	2009	2010	2011	2012	2013	2014	2015
Azerbaijan					1,366	359		598	
Afghanistan	21,887	50,839	37,641	27,571	27,915	15,968	35,282	21,052	49,048
Uzbekistan			1,789		2,421	15,731	2,151		2,230
Australia	12,463	3,809	2,178						
Kazakhstan			5,936			1,900			
South Korea								3,325	
China	372,387	490,492	379,673	549,186	883,138	1329,692	1836,353	1526,111	1558,603
Turkmenistan			11,054	9,831	53,789				
Pakistan			502		10,107	26,854	12,867	6,468	
Myanmar		221							
Mongolia			1,985			250			
Russia				1,393	13,980		237	262	35,411

Table 2. Cumulative total value of Japanese licorice imports, in 1,000 yen, from its major trading partners (2007–2015).

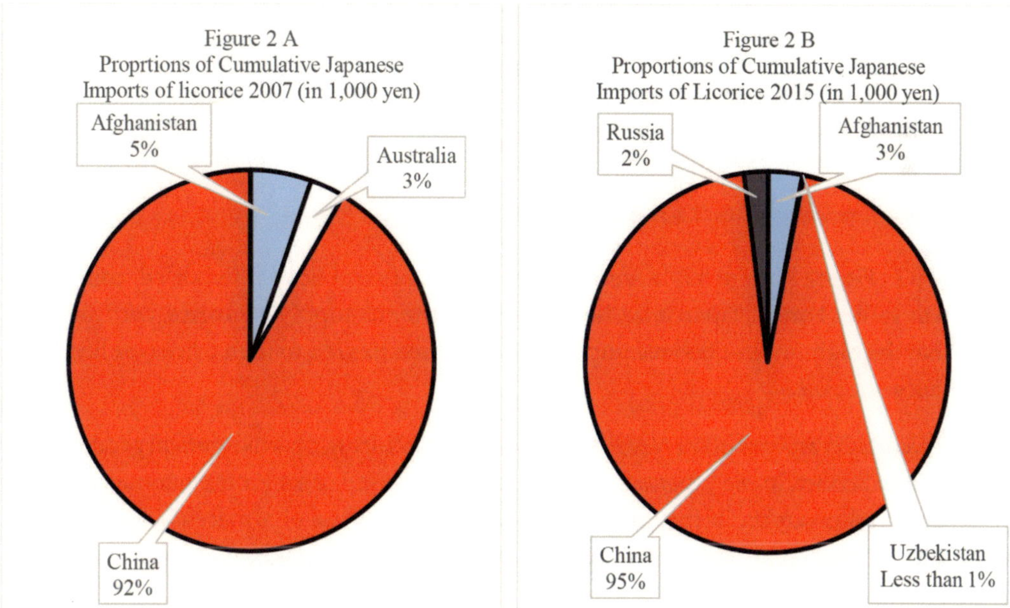

Figure 2. (A) Proportion of cumulative Japanese imports of licorice 2007 (in 1,000 yen). (B) Proportion of cumulative Japanese imports of licorice 2015 (in 1,000 yen).

However, closer investigation reveals a problem that Japan may face in the near future.

Figure 3 shows the import price of Chinese licorice per kilogram (in 1,000 yen).[3] These data show that the import price of licorice from China has been increasing for several years. In particular, the dramatic rise in the price of imported Chinese licorice after 2012 is remarkable, with the price in 2015 being nearly three times that in 2007.

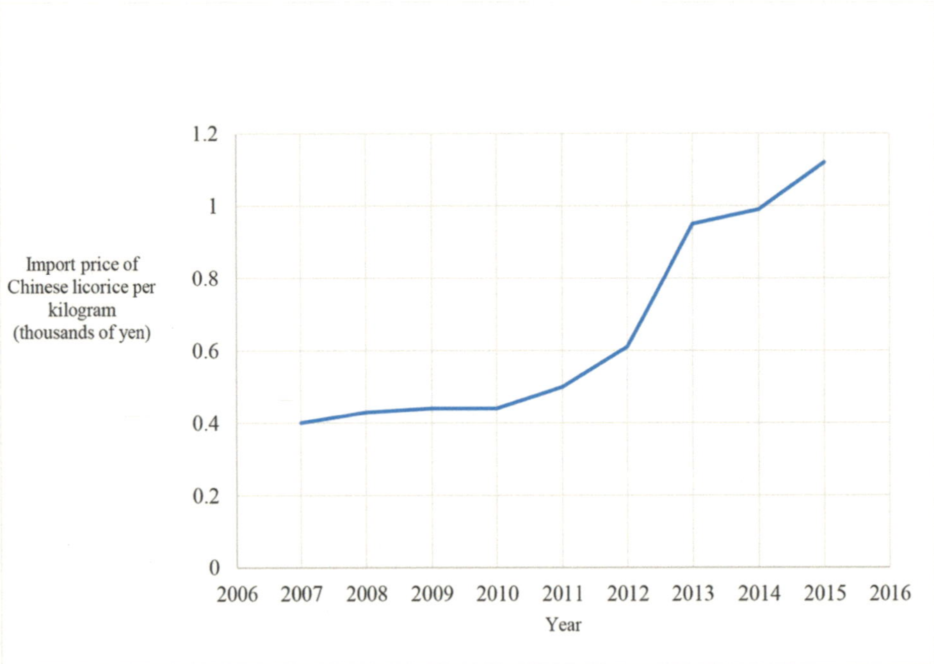

Figure 3. Trend in the import price of Chinese licorice (2007–2015).

As shown in **Figure 3**, there has been an increase in the price of licorice imported from China. As seen in **Tables 1** and **2**, Japan relies heavily on China for its supply of licorice, with the result being that the high price of licorice imported from China has led to high prices for licorice in the Japanese market.

Because licorice is an important raw material for manufacturing pharmaceutical products, the high price of licorice in the Japanese market causes increased costs for the manufacturing of pharmaceutical products. If this high price continues, then the pharmaceutical industry in Japan may be affected by budget constraints in the production of medical products containing licorice.

[3] **Figure 3** is derived from Trade Statistics of Japan conducted by the Japanese Ministry of Finance (http://www.customs.go.jp/toukei/srch/index.htm?M=01&P=0) [Accessed: 2016-09-17]. Import prices in **Figure 3** are calculated as cumulative amount spent on Japanese imports of licorice from China in **Table 2** divided by the cumulative total volume of Japanese import of licorice from China in **Table 1**. For detail, we amend per-unit data in **Table 1** from tons to kilograms.

http://dx.doi.org/10.5772/66514

3. Basic economic concepts

3.1. Economics terms used

As discussed in the previous section, China is the most important source of licorice for the Japanese market. In addition, the price of licorice from China has been increasing in recent years. In this section, we try to understand this situation in economic terms by considering the potential causes for the increasing price of Chinese licorice and its impact on the Japanese market.

We attempt to use basic, rather than highly specialized terminology[4] in this chapter as many of its readers will be experts in pharmacology, but unfamiliar with economics.

In mainstream economics, the price and quantity traded of goods and services are determined mainly by supply and demand. To understand this concept properly, we first introduce definitions of several important economic terms. We refer specifically to reference [5] to define the terms market, quantity demanded, the law of demand, quantity supplied, the law of supply, and market equilibrium. We define these terms as per reference [5] as follows:

A market is defined as "a group of buyers and sellers of a particular good or service."

Quantity demanded is defined as "the amount of the good that buyers are willing and able to purchase."

The law of demand is defined as "the claim that, other things being equal, the quantity demanded of a good falls when the price of the good rises."

Quantity supplied is defined as "the amount of a good that sellers are willing and able to sell."

The law of supply is defined as "the claim that, other things being equal, the quantity supplied of a good rises when the price of the good rises."

Market equilibrium is defined as "a situation in which the market price has reached the level at which quantity supplied equals quantity demanded."

Figure 4[5] summarizes the definitions above. The curves here are referred to as the demand curve and the supply curve of a good.[6] We can see that the demand curve and the supply curve are downward-sloping and upward-sloping, respectively. The shapes of the curves are due to the aforementioned laws of demand and supply.

As seen in **Figure 4**, there is a point at which the demand curve and the supply curve intersect. This intersection is the graphical representation of the market equilibrium. The

---

[4] The discussion in Section 3 derives primarily from Ref. [5].

[5] **Figure 4** is prepared by the author on the basis of Ref. [5].

[6] In Ref. [5], the demand and supply schedules are determined as a graph of the relationship between the price of a good and the quantity demanded and a graph of the relationship between the price of a good and the quantity supplied, respectively. In **Figure 4**, a good's price and quantity traded are indicated on the vertical and horizontal axes, respectively. The demand schedule, supply schedule, equilibrium, price at equilibrium, and quantity at equilibrium are labeled D, S, E, Pe, and Qe, respectively.

actions of buyers and sellers naturally move markets toward the equilibrium of supply and demand [5].[7]

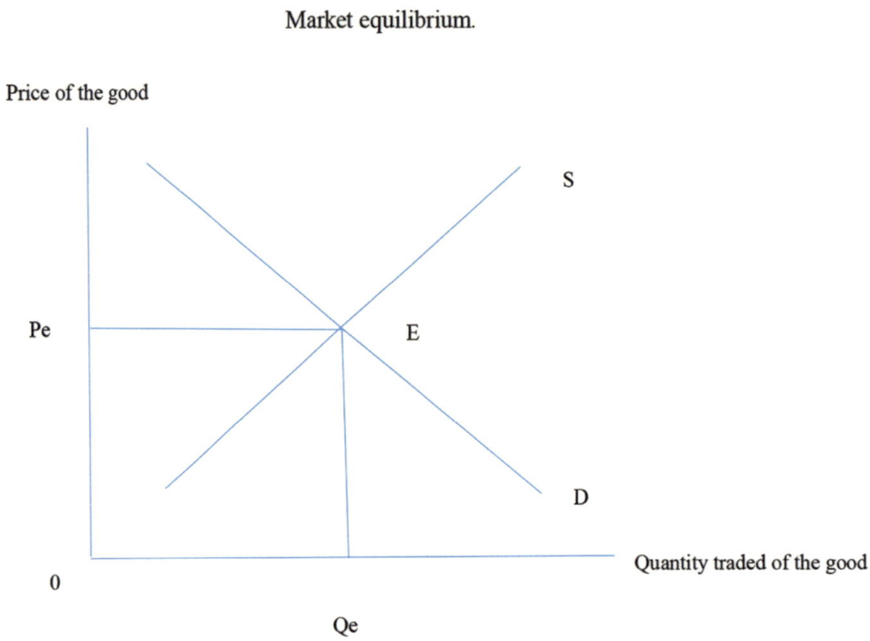

Figure 4. Market equilibrium.

3.2. Shifts of the demand and supply curves

Up to this point, we have understood that the price and quantity traded of a good are determined by its market equilibrium. However, as mentioned in the definitions of the laws of demand and supply, this is true if and only if all factors other than the price and quantity traded of the good are held constant. This is unrealistic because there are numerous factors affecting a good's price and traded quantity [5].

In this subsection, therefore, we try to understand a case when the aforementioned assumption is relaxed.

As described in reference [5], if something happens to alter the quantity demanded at any given price, then this is expressed through a shift of the demand curve. Specifically, any change that increases the quantity demanded at every price shifts the demand curve to the right. This shift is due to factors other than price that may increase the consumers' willingness to consume the good at any given price. Buyers now want to purchase a larger quantity of the good, with the opposite holding true as well.

[7] In the short run, there are possibilities to have price and quantity traded of the good at points other than the market equilibrium. However, these occurrences are often accompanied by excess demand and supply, and market settles at equilibrium in the long run. For a more detailed description, see Ref. [5].

http://dx.doi.org/10.5772/66514

To help understand how shifts in the demand curve occur, below we refer to three representative examples of the factors used in economics as presented in reference [5].

The first factor relating to demand for a good is income. Suppose that consumers' incomes fall and they have less money to spend, as a result, consumers' consumption of a good will be lower at a given price. Conversely, if consumers' incomes rise, then they take the opposite action.

The second factor relating to demand for a good is the price of related goods. When consumers purchase something, they often compare its price to that of its substitutes (i.e., ice cream and frozen yogurt). If the price of a substitute is cheaper, then the consumers may choose to buy the substitute and vice versa.

A third factor relating to demand for a good is the number of buyers. If the number of consumers in the market increases, then the quantity demanded in the market will increase at any given price. Conversely, if some consumers stop consuming the good, the quantity demanded will decrease.

In addition to the factors discussed above, public policy makers can also influence the quantity demanded. One way to influence demand is to impose a tax. If policy makers consider consumption of a good to be unsuitable (e.g., cigarettes), then they may impose a tax on that product on for the purpose of raising its price [5].

The shift in the demand curve discussed above is depicted in **Figure 5**.[8] We can see that the demand curve can shift to the right or to the left. As shown in the figure, the former leads to an increase in quantity demanded while the latter leads to a decrease in quantity demanded [5].

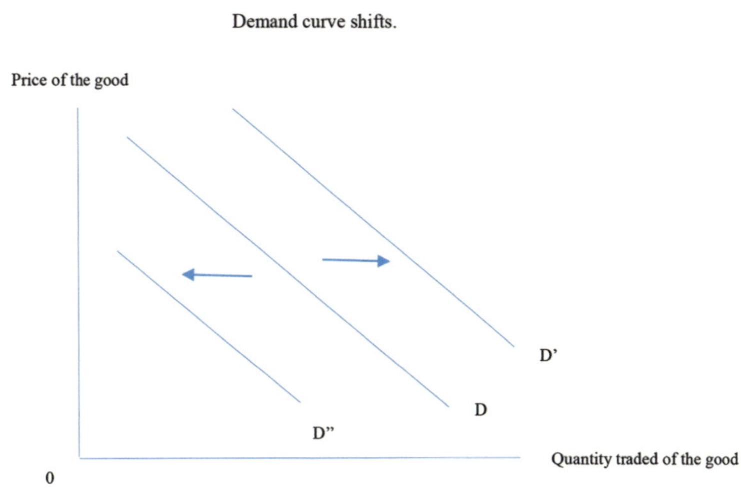

Figure 5. Demand curve shifts.

[8] **Figure 5** is drawn from Ref. [5]. Price and quantity traded of the good are indicated on the vertical and horizontal axes, respectively. The initial demand schedule, a rightward shift, and a leftward shift are labeled D, D', and D", respectively.

In reference [5], if something occurs that alters the quantity supplied at any given price, then the supply curve is shifted. This shift is due to the following factors. If there are factors other than price that increase the suppliers' willingness to supply the good at any given price, then sellers are willing to produce a larger quantity, and the supply curve shifts to the right, with the opposite also holding true.

We also refer to three representative examples of the economic concepts presented in reference [5].

The first factor determining the supply of the good is its input price. To produce the good, suppliers incur costs such as material and labor costs. If these costs increase, then the suppliers' profit from selling the good at the given price will decrease, thus lowering the quantity supplied.

The second factor to consider is technology. If the technology for turning inputs into a final product is improved (e.g., new machinery or methods are developed and fewer inputs and time are required to produce a given quantity of the good), production costs will be reduced, helping to increase supply.

A third factor relating to the supply of a good is the number of sellers. If the number of sellers in a market increases (i.e., new suppliers enter the market), then the quantity supplied in the market will be increased.

Similar to the case of the demand curve, public policy makers can also influence the quantity of the good supplied. This can be accomplished in several ways, including through regulations. Policy makers regulate the supply of the product when they consider the supply of the good to be socially undesirable [5].

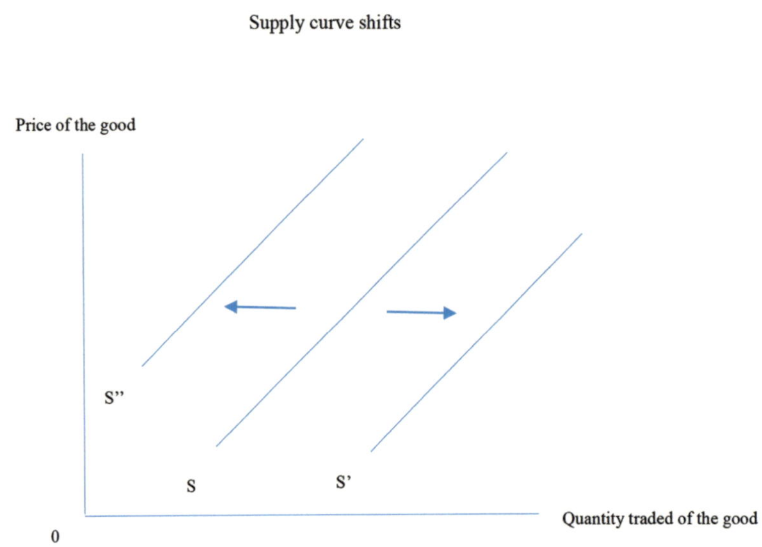

Figure 6. Supply curve shifts.

The shift in the supply curve discussed above is depicted in **Figure 6**. As in the case of the demand curve, the supply curve can shift to the right or to the left. As shown in this figure, the former leads to an increase in quantity supplied while the latter leads to a decrease in the quantity supplied [5].[9]

In this subsection, we referred to reference [5] to describe the basic terms and concepts of economics. In economic market analysis, the price and quantity traded of a good are determined by its market equilibrium (i.e., the point where demand and supply meet). In addition, factors other than price may shift the demand and supply of a product. We also gave examples of the factors influencing demand and supply in reference [5]. However, there are numerous other factors affecting the demand and supply of a good.

4. Potential causes of the high price of imported Chinese licorice

Our aim in this section is to understand the recent high prices of imported Chinese licorice using the economic concepts explained in the previous section. More specifically, we consider the potential causes of the high price of Chinese licorice in Japan and how it can be understood in economic terms by looking at changes in its supply and demand.

One of the potential major causes of the high price of Chinese licorice is the fluctuation of the exchange rate between the Japanese yen and the Chinese yuan. In the period 2007–2015, the value of the Japanese yen fell against Chinese yuan. This caused Chinese products to become more expensive in Japan. Viewed in the context of the market analysis from Section 3, we find that from the suppliers' point of view, there has been an increase in their input costs (i.e., a leftward shift of the supply curve). However, it is simplistic to assume that the high price of Chinese licorice in Japan is solely a result of the depreciation of Japanese yen. There are, in fact, several other matters that can potentially affect the price and trading volume of Chinese licorice in the Japanese market.

As was mentioned before, licorice is one of the most commonly used herbal medicines in the production of pharmaceutical products [2]. In recent years, the production of pharmaceutical products using licorice as a raw material has increased steadily. **Figure 7** shows the value (in millions of yen) of pharmaceutical production using licorice as a raw material in Japan in the period 2007–2014.[10]

As seen in **Figure 7**, the value of the pharmaceutical production using licorice as a raw material in Japan in this period increased. This is likely due to the growing need for pharmaceutical products in the Japanese medical field. This trend can be understood from an economic point of view in the following manner. This growing need for pharmaceutical products increases

[9] **Figure 6** originates from Ref. [5]. In this figure, price and quantity traded of the good are indicated on the vertical and horizontal axes, respectively. The initial supply schedule, a rightward shift, and a leftward shift are labeled S, S', and S'', respectively.

[10] **Figure 7** is prepared by the author from the statistics of production by pharmaceutical industry conducted by the Japanese Ministry of Health, Labour and Welfare (http://www.mhlw.go.jp/toukei/list/105-1.html) [Accessed: 2016-09-17]. Data limitations prevent us from introducing 2015 data.

demand for certain materials (e.g., Chinese licorice). Applying this to the market analysis discussed in Section 3, we find an increase in the demand for Chinese licorice, causing the demand curve to shift to the right.

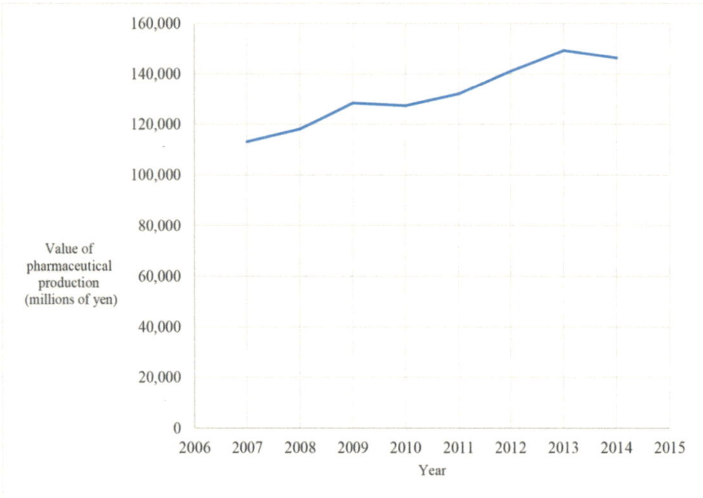

Figure 7. Trend in the value of pharmaceutical production using licorice in Japan (2007–2014).

By examining the supply of licorice in China, we find certain factors leading to the increased price. So far, almost all licorice produced in China involves its native strains, as cultivation methods for licorice are not widely established in China [1]. As with natural resources, the amount is limited, and continuous collection causes their depletion. In addition, excessive harvesting can also cause desertification of that area [3]. To prevent the depletion of native licorice and the destruction associated with its harvest, the Chinese government began to restrict the harvest of native licorice in 1984. These restrictions did not apply to three northern regions (the province of Gansu and the two autonomous regions of Neimenggu and Ningxia) [1]. These restrictions were tightened in 2000 [1]. This reduced the supply of native licorice as a herbal medicine in China. Using the market analysis from Section 3, we find a leftward shift of the supply curve of Chinese licorice.

There are other issues that had negative impacts on the supply of Chinese licorice. For example, China has recently been experiencing rapid economic growth, which may bring about an increase in the price of commodities, including licorice. Moreover, Chinese economic growth also increases the labor costs of licorice production. Labor costs are considered part of the input price of licorice. As a result, the input costs of licorice become more expensive at any given price. From the market analysis in Section 3, there is a leftward shift of the supply curve.

As discussed above, there are several issues affecting the supply and demand of Chinese licorice. We now try to simulate the price and quantity traded of Chinese licorice in the Japanese market by examining the changes in its demand and supply. As noted in the discussion of

http://dx.doi.org/10.5772/66514

economic concepts, the price and amount traded of a product are generally determined by its supply and demand [5]. We also discussed how supply and demand are potentially affected by factors such as the growing needs of pharmaceutical producers, restrictions on the harvesting of licorice, and increases in labor costs. The current situation for Chinese licorice in Japan can be visualized in **Figure 8**, where market equilibrium is determined by a demand curve with a rightward shift and a supply curve with a leftward shift.[11]

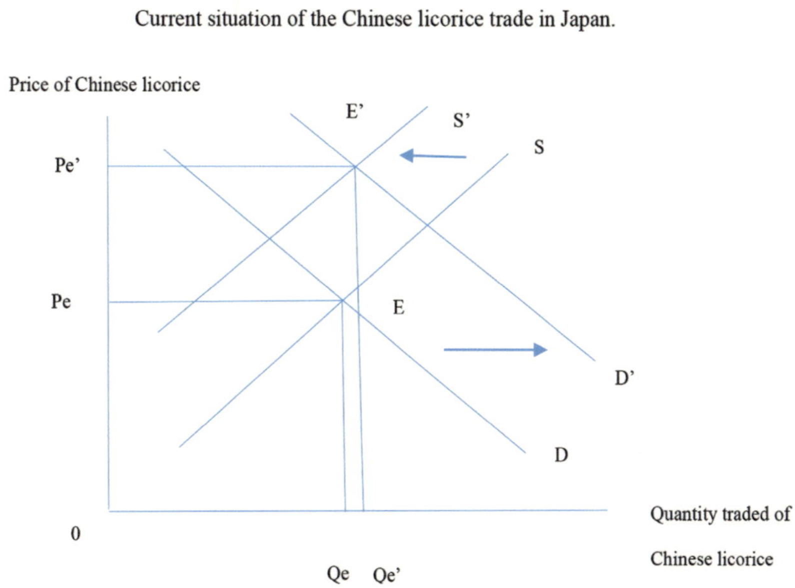

Figure 8. Current situation of the Chinese licorice trade in Japan.

As seen in **Figure 8**, at the new equilibrium (E'), the price of licorice is higher than it was previously considered. There is a possibility that this simulation in our market analysis describes the recent rise in the price of Chinese licorice in the Japanese market.[12]

5. Necessity of alternative sources of supply

As was discussed in the previous section, the recent increase in the price of Chinese licorice in the Japanese market is considered to be due to a combined effect of an increase in its demand

---

[11] **Figure 8** presents Japanese demand and supply of Chinese licorice following [5]. The price and quantity traded of Chinese licorice are indicated on the vertical and horizontal axes, respectively. The initial demand schedule, a rightward shift in demand, the initial supply schedule, a leftward shift in the supply schedule, the equilibrium, the equilibrium price, the equilibrium quantity, the new equilibrium, the new equilibrium price, and the new equilibrium quantity are labeled D, D', S, S', E, Pe, Qe, E', Pe', and Qe', respectively.

[12] As in **Figure 8**, the rightward shift of the demand schedule and the leftward shift of the supply schedule counteract the respective effects on quantity traded. Hence, changes in quantity traded depend on the comparative strength of influences from demand and supply.

and decrease in its supply. Although the depreciation of the Japanese yen may be improved by changes in each country's economic situation, a decrease in the harvest of native licorice cannot be improved without taking precautionary measures. Leaving the market could potentially cause further increases in the price and a reduction of trading volume. Eventually, the trade of licorice in the Japanese market may become difficult to sustain.

To prevent such a situation, the price and trading volume of licorice must be maintained by increasing its supply. In this section, we discuss attempts to establish licorice cultivation methods, which could potentially serve as a supply source of an alternative to native Chinese licorice. If cultivated licorice can be used in Japanese pharmaceutical products in the same way as its native strains, then decreases in the supply of native licorice could be offset with cultivated licorice.

Figure 9 visualizes the situation described above.[13]

As shown in **Figure 9**, due to the combined effect of an increase in demand and a decrease in supply, the current equilibrium condition of Chinese licorice in the Japanese market is considered to be at *E′*. Utilizing cultivated licorice as an alternative to native licorice could help shift the supply curve to the right, leading to an equilibrium point at *E″*. At *E″*, the price of licorice will be lower than in the previous situation (i.e., price at the equilibrium (*E′*)).

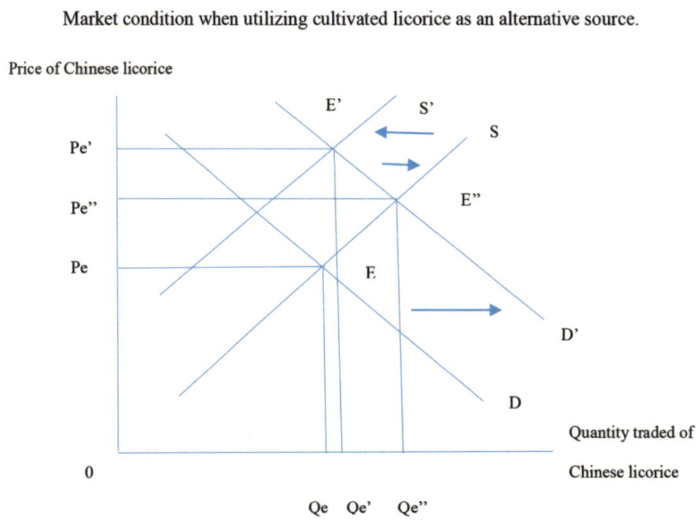

Figure 9. Market condition when utilizing cultivated licorice as an alternative source.

[13] Drawn from Ref. [5], **Figure 9** simulates Japanese demand and supply for licorice when cultivated licorice becomes an alternative. The price and quantity traded are indicated on the vertical and horizontal axes, respectively. The initial demand schedule, a rightward shift, the initial supply schedule, a leftward shift, initial equilibrium price and quantity, and new equilibrium price and quantity are labeled D, D′, S, S′, E, Pe, Qe, E′, Pe′, and Qe′, respectively. In addition, equilibriums following the introduction of cultivated licorice, the third equilibrium price, and the third equilibrium quantity are labeled E", Pe", and Qe", respectively.

http://dx.doi.org/10.5772/66514

However, using cultivated licorice as an alternative to native Chinese licorice is not an easy task. This is because the amount of cultivated licorice needed as an ingredient in Japanese pharmaceutical products is often different from that of native licorice. More specifically, the glycyrrhizin content (an ingredient contained in licorice root) of cultivated licorice is often lower than that of native licorice [1].

Because of this, the content of pharmaceutical products produced using cultivated licorice must conform to the standards of official compendiums such as the Japanese Pharmacopoeia XIV (JP XIV)[14] (e.g., see Ref. [1]).

A number of groups are performing research on the production of cultivated licorice that can be used in pharmaceutical products in Japan.

Reference [6] reports an investigation of the quality variation of the licorice in the Japanese market in the period 1986–2000. The main contribution of this investigation was to propose a method of distinguishing the different types of Chinese licorice. More specifically, during the investigation period, the average glycyrrhizin content of Dongbei-Gancao, a type of licorice mainly traded in the Japanese market, was found to be higher than that of a different type of licorice, Xibei-Gancao. On the other hand, the root specific gravity of Dongbei-Gancao is often lower than that of Xibei-Gancao. The investigation also found that some Dongbei-Gancao has high root specific gravity, which is not consistent with the aforementioned characteristic of Dongbei-Gancao. The investigation suggests that the licorice that was thought to be Dongbei-Gancao seems to correspond to Ditou-Gancao, which is a Chinese licorice different from both the Dongbei and Xibei types.

Reference [7] reports a study of the cultivation of *Glycyrrhiza uralensis* (the scientific names of one type of licorice) in the eastern region of Neimenggu (Inner Mongolia). In this study, seeds of *G. uralensis* were sown in May 1998 and its seedling roots were transplanted to the field the following May. It was found that the glycyrrhizin content of 4-year-old lateral root newly grown from the transplanted seedling taproot exceeds the Japanese Pharmacopoeia XIV standard. However, the study concludes that utilizing the cultivated licorice as a substitute for the native licorice traded in the Japanese market is still difficult, because even though the glycyrrhizin content of the cultivated licorice satisfies JP XIV, it is still lower than that of the native licorice currently traded in the Japanese market. The study emphasizes the necessity of improvements in the selection of seedlings and cultivation methods.

In reference [3], the feasibility of the medicinal use of cultivated licorice was tested by comparing the licorice roots cultivated in eastern Neimenggu and that used in medical applications. According to this study, the 4-year-old adventitious licorice roots cultivated in eastern Neimenggu may be a suitable substitute for licorice conforming to JP XIV.

Attempts are also being made to cultivate licorice in Japan. In reference [8], a comparative study of 10 types of licorice strains cultivated in the Kyoto Herbal Garden of Takeda Pharma-

[14] JP XIV standards appear in the 14th edition of the Japanese Pharmacopoeia, which was published to regulate the properties and quality of drugs by the Japanese Minister of Health, Labor and Welfare after consultation with the Pharmaceutical Affairs and Food Sanitation Council. The 17th edition is the latest version. For details, see http://www.mhlw.go.jp/stf/seisakunitsuite/bunya/0000066597.html [Accessed: 2016-09-17].

ceutical Co. Ltd. was undertaken to understand the differences of the features of licorice of different origins. According to this latter study, the 10 types of licorice belong to either the Chinese or the Kazakhstani types. These types show some differences, namely the glycyrrhizin content of Chinese type is higher than that of Kazakhstani type.

In reference [4], a study of the cultivation of licorice in Inner Mongolia was conducted. This study aimed to confirm the origin of the plant by comparing their cultivated strain to native strains in the Xinjiang Uygur Autonomous Region of China.[15] The study concludes that their cultivated strain of licorice is most likely the *G. uralensis*, which is the main raw material of licorice used in Japan.

In reference [9], a study investigated the use of cultivated licorice in Inner Mongolia as a method to compensate for the reduced supply of native licorice. Specifically, the chemical and pharmaceutical properties of cultivated licorice root and those of licorice prepared from its native plant were compared. In this study, boiled water extracts of cultivated and native licorice were found to have similar antispasmodic effect on carbachol-induced contraction in mice jejunum.[16] Moreover, the glycycoumarin content (one of the components contained in licorice) of boiled water extract of 4-year-old cultivated root and that of native licorice was also found to be similar. Thus, the study in reference [9] concluded that the cultivated licorice root could be considered an adequate substitute in the face of restrictions on the harvest of native licorice.

Some researchers are attempting to use the cultivation of licorice to prevent desertification, mainly in Mongolia. This is referred to as high-value-added greening, since it is effective in both providing a supply of licorice and combatting desertification. In reference [10], desertification is explained as an environmental problem caused by both natural environmental phenomena, such as irregular precipitation and the lowering of the ground water level, and anthropogenic causes such as overharvesting of native plants.

Many of the studies referenced here take advantage of greening soil materials (GSMs). In reference [11], GSMs are a mixture of sand and compost that can be inexpensively and easily applied to the ground. This material contains more water than ordinary soils and, therefore, can be thought of as a simple self-watering system that does not require artificial water supplies.

There have been various reports on the effect of using GSMs to cultivate licorice.

To prevent desertification, in reference [10], licorice was experimentally planted in arid areas of Mongolia. In this experiment, GSMs were used for planting licorice. As GSMs have more than 10 times the water and nutrient-holding capacity in comparison with desert ground, a correlation between the survival ratio of licorice and GSMs was demonstrated (i.e., a positive relationship between the amount of water in GSMs and the survival ratio of licorice).

Reference [11] reports field agricultural experiments conducted in areas where licorice did not grow naturally. In this experiment, researchers concluded that a larger volume of GSMs could

---

[15] Native strains of licorice in the latter area are *Glycyrrhiza inflata, G. glabra, and G. uralensis*.

[16] Carbachol is a kind of medicine (cholinergic agent).

http://dx.doi.org/10.5772/66514

maintain the survival rate for licorice higher than smaller types. In other words, GSMs are helpful in increasing the survival rate of licorice.

In reference [12], a geo-environmental and climate survey was conducted to investigate the environmental conditions in the licorice-habitat area. In this study as well, GSMs were used experimentally to plant licorice in arid Mongolian land. This experiment reached several conclusions. First, there was a great difference between the licorice habitat and non-habitat areas in terms of the amount of water in the ground. Specifically, at points deeper than 20 cm below the surface, the water content was higher in the habitat area of licorice than in non-habitat areas. Second, covering the ground surface with vinyl-mulching sheets helps licorice to survive by maintaining a high water content. Third, GSMs help licorice to survive by maintaining a high water content. Fourth, licorice can survive if soil water content of at least 8% is maintained.

In reference [13], agricultural experiments were conducted in sandy ground to simulate arid regions and non-habitat regions of licorice in Mongolia, using GSMs to establish suitable soil water and calcium conditions, setting up outer layer processing for the survival and growth of licorice. In this experiment, some beneficial results were obtained. Notably, the active ingredient content of the cultivated licorice root tended to rise when using GSMs whose available moisture was three to 10 times higher than that in Mongolian soils.

In reference [14], the five bioactive components of licorice (liquiritin, liquiritigenin, glycyrrhizin, isoliquiritin, and isoliquiritigenin) were examined using four types of licorice grown in four distinct environments in Northern China during 2010–2011. This study explored how the five bioactive components are affected by various factors, such as climate (i.e., an increase in the duration of sunshine increases glycyrrhizin while declining rainfall promotes the accumulation of liquiritigenin and isoliquiritigenin).

As was discussed in this section, the effects of a decrease in the harvest of native Chinese licorice cannot be underestimated as it has the potential to cause further price increases and reductions in trading volume. Eventually, the trading of licorice in the Japanese market may become difficult to sustain.

To prevent such a situation, the price and trading volume of licorice must be maintained by increasing its supply. One of the potential solutions is to establish cultivation methods for licorice.

However, using cultivated licorice as an alternative supply source is not an easy task, since the amounts of active ingredients in cultivated licorice are often different from those in the native licorice used for pharmaceutical products in Japan [1].

As noted in this section, a number of groups are attempting to establish cultivation methods for licorice that can be used in the pharmaceutical industry in Japan.

However, to conclude that the quality of cultivated licorice is equivalent to that of native licorice, more demonstrations are required. More specifically, further studies are needed to devise methods for increasing the glycyrrhizin content of cultivated licorice.

6. Conclusion

Recent years have seen changes in the trade of licorice between Japan and China. Specifically, the import price of Chinese licorice has been steadily increasing. As the high price of Chinese licorice is expected to continue, the use of Chinese licorice in Japan will be constrained.

Unlike in pharmacological studies, here we investigated at data such as the price and trading volume between China and Japan to analyze the licorice market from an economic perspective. So far, publications analyzing licorice by incorporating economic concepts is rare. Our study constitutes a novel analysis of trends in the licorice market.

This study investigated changes in the supply, demand, and quantity traded of licorice. We concluded that the recent high price of Chinese licorice in Japan is likely due to the combined effect of an increase in demand and a decrease in supply.

To alleviate this situation, the price and quantity traded of licorice must be maintained by increasing its supply.

As the number of native strains in China is limited, its supply is unlikely to increase.

One way to increase the supply of licorice without relying on native Chinese strains is to establish methods of licorice cultivation. If cultivated licorice can be used to manufacture pharmaceutical products in the same way as native strains, then cultivated licorice will serve as a useful alternative supply source to compensate for the decrease in the supply of native strains.

However, to achieve this, there are many problems that must be solved, and a great deal of future research will be necessary.

Acknowledgements

I am grateful for the special grant from the Miyata Research Scholarship in fiscal year 2016 that supported this research. I also received valuable comments from an editor.

Author details

Ryusuke Oishi

Address all correspondence to: r-o@meikai.ac.jp

Meikai University, Faculty of Economics, Urayasu, Japan

References

[1] Yamamoto Y, Tani T. Field study and pharmaceutical evaluation of *Glycyrrhiza uralensis* roots cultivated in China. Journal of Traditional Medicines. 2005;22(Suppl 1):86–97.

[2] Hayashi H, Sudo H. Economic importance of licorice. Plant Biotechnology. 2009;26(1): 101–104. DOI: 10.5511/plantbiotechnology.26.101

[3] Yamamoto Y, Majima T, Saiki I, Tani T. Pharmaceutical evaluation of *Glycyrrhiza uralensis* roots cultivated in eastern Nei-Meng-Gu of China. Biological and Pharmaceutical Bulletin. 2003;26(8):1144–1149. DOI: 10.1248/bpb.26.1144

[4] Yamamoto Y, Tani T. Brief survey of Glycyrrhiza plant resources in Xinjiang, China. Journal of Traditional Medicines. 2006;23(1):27–35. DOI: 10.11339/jtm.23.27

[5] Mankiw NG. Principles of Economics. 7th ed. Stanford: Cengage Learning; 2014.

[6] Yamamoto Y, Tani T. Evaluation of glycyrrhizin variation in Gancao collected from 1986 to 2000 at drug markets in Japan and discrimination of Daitou-Gancao and Dongbei-Gancao. Journal of Traditional Medicines. 2001;18:197–202.

[7] Yamamoto Y, Tani T. Growth and glycyrrhizin contents in *Glycyrrhiza uralensis* roots cultivated for four years in eastern Nei-Meng-gu of China. Journal of Traditional Medicines. 2002;19:87–92.

[8] Hayashi H, Inoue K, Ozaki K, Watanabe H. Comparative analysis of ten strains of *Glycyrrhiza uralensis* cultivated in Japan. Biological and Pharmaceutical Bulletin. 2005;28(6):1113–1116. DOI: 10.1248/bpb.28.1113

[9] Nagai H, Yamamoto Y, Sato Y, Akao T, Tani T. Pharmaceutical evaluation of cultivated *Glycyrrhiza uralensis* roots in composition of their antispasmodic activity and glycycoumarin content with those of licorice. Biological and Pharmaceutical Bulletin. 2006;29(12):2442–2445. DOI: 10.1248/bpb.29.2442

[10] Furukawa Z, Yasufuku N, Omine K, Marui A, Kameoka R, Mandakh B, Tuvsintogotokh I. Conditions of developed greening soil materials (GSM) for survival of licorice and combating desertification. Japanese Geotechnical Society Special Publication. 2015;1(4): 25–29. DOI: 10.3208/jgssp.JPN-33

[11] Furukawa Z, Yasufuku N, Omine K, Marui A, Kameoka R, Tuvshintogtokh I, Mandakh B, Bat-Eneral B, Yeruult Y. Setting and geo-environmental conditions of developed greening soil materials (GSM) for cultivating licorice (*Glycyrrhiza uralensis* fisch.) in Mongolian arid region. Journal of Arid Land Studies. 2015;25(3):105–108. DOI: 10.14976/jals.25.3_105

[12] Kameoka R, Yasufuku N, Omine K, Murai A, Furukawa Z, Tuvshintogtokh I, Mandakh B, Bat-Eneral B, Yeruult Y. Developing licorice planting techniques with cultural

experiments focused on the water conditions of green soil materials. Journal of Arid land Studies. 2015;25(3):97–100. DOI: 10.14976/jals.25.3_97

[13] Furukawa Z, Yasufuku N, Kameoka R. A study on effects and functions of developed greening soil materials (GSM) for combining desertification. Japanese Geotechnical Society Special Publication. 2015;2(56):1928–1933. DOI: 10.3208/jgssp.JPN-052

[14] Yu F, Wang Q, Wei S, Wang D, Fang Y, Liu F, Zhao Z, Hou J, Wang W. Effect of genotype and environment on five bioactive components of cultivated licorice (*Glycyrrhiza uralensis*) populations in northern China. Biological and Pharmaceutical Bulletin. 2015;38(1):75–81. DOI: 10.1248/bpb.b14-00574

Section 2

Structural-Activity Relationship of Licorice Phenolics

Chapter 4

Licorice as a Resource for Pharmacologically Active Phenolic Substances: Antioxidant and Antimicrobial Effects

Tsutomu Hatano, Eerdunbayaer, Yanmei Cui,
Teruo Kuroda and Yuuki Shimozu

Additional information is available at the end of the chapter

http://dx.doi.org/10.5772/66419

Abstract

The findings from our studies on licorice phenolics are summarized here. The following types of flavonoids, i.e., flavones, flavonols, flavanones, chalcones, isoflavones, isoflavanones, isoflavans, 3-arylcoumarins, coumestans, pterocarpans, 2-benzyldihydrobenzofuran-3-ones, benzyl phenyl ketones, 2-arylbenzofurans, and others, were identified by the structural studies. Among them, licochalcone A (chalcone), isolicoflavonol (flavonol), glycycoumarin (3-arylcoumarin), and glycyrrhisoflavone (isoflavone) displayed antihuman immunodeficiency virus effects, and also 8-(γ,γ-dimethylallyl)-wighteone (isoflavone) and 3′-(γ,γ-dimethylallyl)-kievitone (isoflavanone) showed potent antibacterial effects on methicillin-resistant *Staphylococcus aureus* (MRSA) strains. Licoricidin (isoflavan) suppressed the oxacillin resistance of the MRSA strains noticeably. Effects of phenolics with related structures isolated from *Psoralea corylifolia* were also examined, and bakuchiol (meroterpene), isobavachalcone, and corylifol B (chalcones) also showed potent effects on MRSA strains. Some licorice phenolics such as licoricidin (isoflavan), 8-(γ,γ-dimethylallyl)-wighteone (isoflavone), and gancaonin I (2-arylbenzofuran) also showed potent antibacterial effects on vancomycin-resistant *Enterococcus* (VRE) strains. The potency of the effects largely depended on their structures including the lipophilic prenyl or related substituents and also phenolic hydroxyl groups. Inhibitory effects of licorice phenolics on oxidative enzymes, in addition to their radical-scavenging effects, are also shown. The methods used in the structural studies and high-performance liquid chromatographic analysis of licorice extracts are described shortly, too.

Keywords: licorice, *Glycyrrhiza*, *Psoralea*, flavonoid, antimicrobial effect

1. Introduction

Licorice (liquorice), the underground portion of *Glycyrrhiza* species, has been used as a remedy for various types of stress, inflammatory diseases, digestive organ disorders, and pain in traditional medicine in Asian and European countries [1, 2]. The main constituent, glycyrrhizin, and the associated aglycone, glycyrrhetinic acid, are also used in modern medicine, whereas the phenolic constituents have been implicated in promoting improved health, particularly with regard to stomach ulcers [2]. Therefore, several research groups have investigated the phenolic constituents of licorice [3] and found that it has beneficial effects for health, including antimicrobial properties [4, 5]. In this chapter, we summarize our studies on phenolic constituents and some of their pharmacological effects, including those linked to drug-resistant bacteria.

2. Findings from our research

Our research on licorice constituents began with an investigation of tannin-like substances in licorice, because tannins and related constituents in medicinal plants have remarkable antioxidant effects, in addition to their fundamental property of binding with proteins, which is related to its various pharmacological effects [6–8]. In fact, licorice extracts of various origins contain tannin-like substances and show protein-binding properties [9]; our additional studies revealed that some phenolic constituents related to flavonoids contribute to this property. Therefore, we investigated these flavonoids and related compounds as discussed below.

2.1. Purification of licorice phenolics

Although classic column chromatography using silica gel has been applied to the separation of phenolic plant constituents, the irreversible adsorption of phenolic constituents (particularly, tannins or tannin-like substances) has limited ability to effectively separate these compounds. Because countercurrent distribution (CCD) does not use solid supports for separation, it can be applied to solve the problem of irreversible adsorption. Thus, centrifugal partition chromatography (CPC) and droplet countercurrent chromatography (DCCC), which were devised as effective methods for CCD, in addition to simple CCD using separatory funnels, were applied to purify the licorice phenolics in our studies. The solvent system chloroform-methanol-water (7:13:8, by volume) was primarily used for the separation of licorice phenolics derived from *Glycyrrhiza inflata* [9, 10] and those derived from *G. uralensis* [11–16] in these CCD processes. Combinations of column chromatography on a silica gel, ODS-gel, and/or polystyrene gel (MCI-gel CHP-20P) with CCD also afforded satisfactory separation [17, 18]. High-performance liquid chromatography (HPLC) was applied for final purification and to establish the purity of the isolated compounds [18, 19]. However, the CCD systems using the solvent systems ethyl acetate-*n*-propanol-water, *n*-hexane-ethanol-water-ethyl acetate, and chloroform-methanol-*n*-propanol-water, in addition to chloroform-methanol-water, were also useful for separating various types of phenolic constituents [17, 20].

2.2. Structural study on licorice phenolics exploring the diversity of their skeletons

Although the structures of aforementioned licorice phenolics were characterized based on the ^{1}H and ^{13}C nuclear magnetic resonance (NMR) spectra, including various 1D and 2D methods, the following spectroscopy methods were also key in establishing the structures. Electron impact mass spectrometry (EI-MS) is a useful method for obtaining structural information using fragment ions [16]. On the other hand, fast-atom bombardment (FAB) and electrospray ionization mass spectrometry (ESI-MS) are applicable to the ionization of phenolics, including phenolic glycosides. Notably, the high-resolution FAB and ESI-MS have been used to determine their molecular formulae [17]. Ultraviolet-visible (UV-Vis) spectroscopy was useful for discriminating between phenolic skeletons even if the ^{1}H NMR spectra were quite similar to each other, as was the case for 3-arylcoumarins and the corresponding isoflavones [16]. Electronic circular dichroism (ECD) spectroscopy was effective not only for identifying the configuration of asymmetric carbons (e.g., those in flavanones, isoflavans, and isoflavanones [9, 15, 17]) in the flavonoid skeletons but also for explaining the spatial relationship between the chromophores in acylated flavonoid glycoside molecules [17]. Based on the data obtained by the aforementioned spectroscopy methods, we uncovered new compound structures and identified known ones isolated from licorice, which can be classified into subgroups based on their structural skeletons as shown in **Table 1**.

As shown in **Table 1**, various types of phenolics have been found in licorice, in addition to the major phenolics (liquiritin, isoliquiritin, and related ones) [21], and their pharmacological properties differ depending on their structures. The strength of the order of the effects also differs depending on the properties examined. Especially, their phenolic hydroxyl and prenyl substituents and also their skeletons related to the molecular flexibility should be considered for their respective properties.

2.3. Properties of licorice phenolics in relation to their health effects

Polyphenols have been linked to antioxidant effects, and some polyphenols such as tannins have protein-binding effects. Interaction of tannins with protein molecules is regarded to be based on hydrophobic interaction and hydrogen bonding and also covalent bonding in some cases [22]. Although some researches focused on the participation of proline residues of proteins in the complexation [23], the modes of complexation are largely dependent on the structures of tannins and proteins/peptides [24–27]. Therefore, further studies using various types of polyphenols should be conducted in order to clarify the complexation. Thus, we examined the binding and antioxidant effects of licorice phenolics.

2.3.1. *Protein-binding and antioxidant effects*

Among the isolated compounds found in large quantities in licorice materials, licochalcone B from Sinkiang (Xinjiang) licorice (mainly collected in the Xinjiang Uyghur Autonomous Region of China) showed the most potent binding activity with proteins, followed by glycyrrhisoflavone from Si-pei (Xi-bei) licorice [9]. Tannins displayed different binding effects depending upon their structures, and licochalcone B and glycyrrhisoflavone (**Figure 1**) showed

Subgroup	Compounds	Origin [a]
Flavones	4′,7-Dihydroxyflavone [9]	*G. inflata*
	3′,4′,7-Trihydroxyflavone [17]	*G. uralensis*
Flavonols	Isolicoflavonol [9], kaempferol-3-*O*-methyl ether [12], licoflavonol, topazolin [16], kaempferol [18], fisetin, glycyrrhiza-flavonol A * [20]	*G. uralensis*
Flavanones	6″-Acetylliquiritin; naringenin [15]; 3′-prenylnaringenin [16]; licorice-glycosides C1 *, C2 *, D1 *, D2 *, and E *; liquiritin apioside [17]; liquiritigenin; liquiritin [21]	*G. uralensis*
Chalcones	Licochalcones A and B [9]	*G. inflata*
	Echinatin [15]; isoliquiritin apioside; licorice glycosides A * and B *; neoisoliquiritin [17]; licochalcone B; tetrahydroxy methoxychalcone * [20]; isoliquiritigenin; isoliquiritin [21]	*G. uralensis*
Isoflavones	Glycyrrhisoflavone * [9]; glisoflavone * [12]; genistein; glicoricone * [14]; 8-(γ,γ-dimethylallyl)-wighteone; gancaonin G; isoangustone A; isowighteone; semilicoisoflavone B [15]; allolicoisoflavone B; 7-*O*-methylluteone; orobol [16]; glycyroside [17]; 5,7-di-*O*-methylluteone *; 6,8-diprenylorobol; formononetin; licoricone [18]; calycosin; glycyrrhiza-isoflavones A *, B *, and C * [20]	*G. uralensis*
Isoflavanones	Glycyrrhisoflavanone * [9], 3′-(γ,γ-dimethylallyl)-kievitone, glicoisoflavanone *, glyasperin F, licoisoflavanone [15], glisoflavanone * [16], glyasperin J, glyasperin J trimethyl ether [19]	*G. uralensis*
Isoflavans	Glyasperin C, glyasperin D, licoricidin, (3*R*)-vestitol [15], (3*R*)-vestitol-7-*O*-glucoside* [17]	*G. uralensis*
3-Arylcoumarins	Glycycoumarin [9], licopyranocoumarin * [11], licoarylcoumarin * [12], glycerin [15], isoglycycoumarin, licofuranocoumarin * [16], 3-(*p*-hydroxyphenyl)-7-methoxycoumarin [18], isolicopyranocoumarin * [20]	*G. uralensis*
Coumestans	Glycyrol, isoglycyrol [15], isotrifoliol * [16], dimethylglycyrol * [18]	*G. uralensis*
Pterocarpans	Demethylhomopterocarpan [19]	*G. uralensis*
2-Benzyldihydro-benzofuran-3-ones	Carpusin [17]	*G. uralensis*
Benzyl phenyl ketones	Glicophenone *, licoriphenone [15]	*G. uralensis*
2-Arylbenzofurans	Licofuranone * [14], licocoumarone [15], gancaonin I [18], glycybenzofuran, 4′-*O*-methylglycybenzofuran *, neoglycybenzofuran * [19]	*G. uralensis*
Benzoic acids	*p*-Hydroxybenzoic acid [20]	*G. uralensis*

[a]The origins were assigned accordingly: *G. uralensis* [Tong-pei licorice and Si-pei (Xi-bei) licorice] and *G. inflata* [Sinkiang (Xinjiang) licorice].
*New compounds.

Table 1. Classification of isolated licorice phenolics.

binding effects more potent than, or comparable to, those of some hydrolyzable tannins such as pedunculagin or corilagin [9, 28].

Then, we examined phenolic radical-scavenging effects on 1,1-diphenyl-2-picrylhydrazyl (DPPH) radicals. Again, licochalcone B displayed the most potent scavenging effects on the DPPH radicals among the examined compounds; licochalcone A showed weaker effects, and isoliquiritigenin and liquiritigenin had negligible effects. The order of potency was as follows:

http://dx.doi.org/10.5772/66419

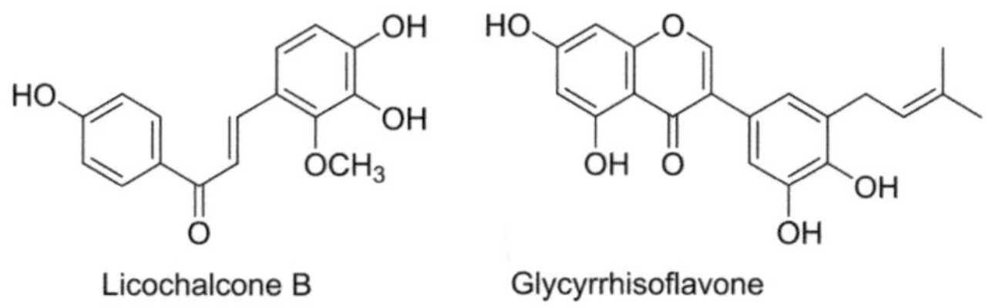

Figure 1. Licorice phenolics with protein-binding activity.

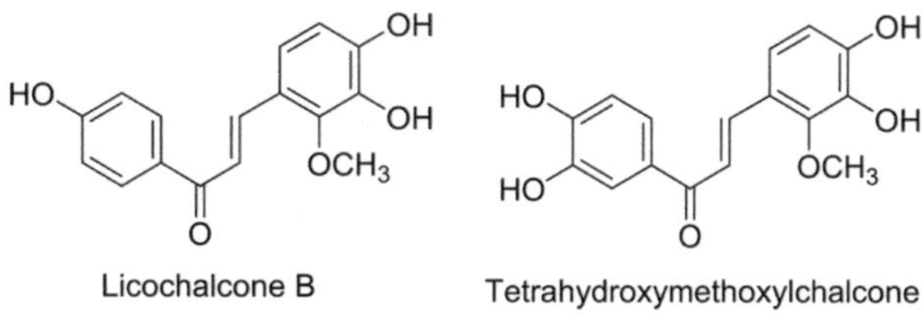

Figure 2. Licorice phenolics forming stable radicals in alkaline DMSO.

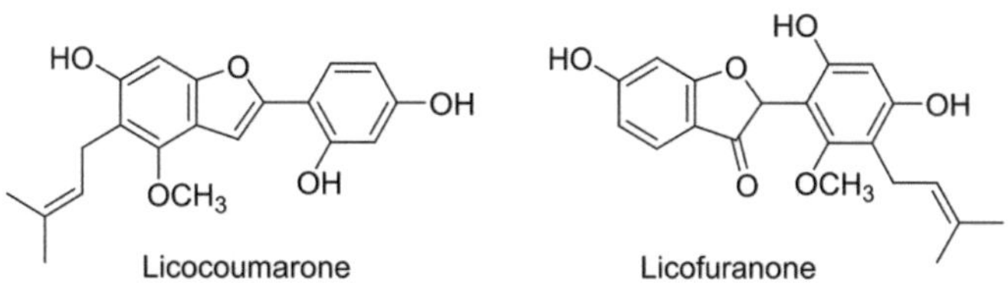

Figure 3. Licorice phenolics with inhibitory effects on oxidative enzymes.

licochalcone B > licochalcone A >> isoliquiritigenin > liquiritigenin. This order of the scavenging effects was the same as that of the reported suppressive effects on lipoxygenase products in arachidonate metabolism [29]. Because stable radical formation was correlated with potent radical-scavenging effects, we examined the formation of radical species from two chalcones, licochalcone B and tetrahydroxy methoxylchalcone (**Figure 2**). As expected, they showed stable electron spin resonance (ESR) signals attributable to their radicals formed by air oxidation in alkaline DMSO solutions [20].

On the other hand, we reported that several licorice phenolics showed inhibitory effects on xanthine oxidase and monoamine oxidase. Licocoumarone, a 2-arylbenzofuran, showed the most potent inhibitory effects on xanthine oxidase, followed by the effects of licochalcone B, licochalcone A, and glycyrrhisoflavone [12]. Two 2-arylbenzofurans, licocoumarone and licofuranone, also showed potent inhibitory effects on monoamine oxidase (**Figure 3**), followed by glycyrrhisoflavone and genistein [14].

The role of xanthine oxidase in the catalysis of the reaction of xanthine into uric acid has been linked to gout and also correlates with the generation of superoxide anion radicals, a reactive oxygen species (ROS). Thus, we examined the effects of licorice phenolics on superoxide generation because ROS have been linked to various kinds of oxidative damage including human organ damage. Licorice phenolics showed suppressive effects on superoxide anion radical generation, both in the enzymatic and nonenzymatic systems examined. In addition to a combination of xanthine oxidase and xanthine (from the enzymatic system), a combination of phenazine methosulfate (PMS) and a reduced form of nicotinamide adenine dinucleotide hydride (NADH) (from the nonenzymatic system) were used for the generating system. On the other hand, detection of the superoxide anion radical was performed using nitroblue tetrazolium and cytochrome c [30]. Three experimental systems composed of the generating and the detection systems indicated that licochalcone B and glycyrrhisoflavone showed potent suppressing effects on superoxide anion radical generation, which are comparable to those of a specific representative flavonoid (quercetin) and a tannin (pedunculagin).

2.3.2. Antihuman immunodeficiency virus effects and suppressive effects on human immunodeficiency virus promoter activity

Further investigation of licorice phenolics revealed that licochalcone A, isolicoflavonol, glycycoumarin, and glycyrrhisoflavone had antiviral effects on human immunodeficiency virus (HIV) (**Figure 4**). HIV causes a "giant cell" in the infected cells OKM-3T (= OKM-1) due to the cytopathic effects of the virus. The aforementioned compounds had inhibitory effects on giant cell formation of a cell line infected with HIV [11, 30]. The mechanisms underlying these antiviral effects may be different from those observed for tannins [31].

Suppressive effects of licorice phenolics on HIV promoters have also been revealed. 12-*O*-Tetradecanoylphorbol-13-acetate (TPA)-induced HIV promoter activity in transfected Jurkat cells was suppressed by glycyrrhisoflavone (isoflavone), tetrahydroxymethoxychalcone, licochalcones A and B (chalcones), glycycoumarin, licopyranocoumarin (3-arylcoumarins), and licocoumarone (2-arylbenzofuran). Although tannins also showed suppressive effects in this experimental system, the effects of licorice phenolics were more potent [32]. On the other hand, licorice phenolics did not show suppressive effects on the cytomegalovirus promoter activity in an analogous experimental system [32].

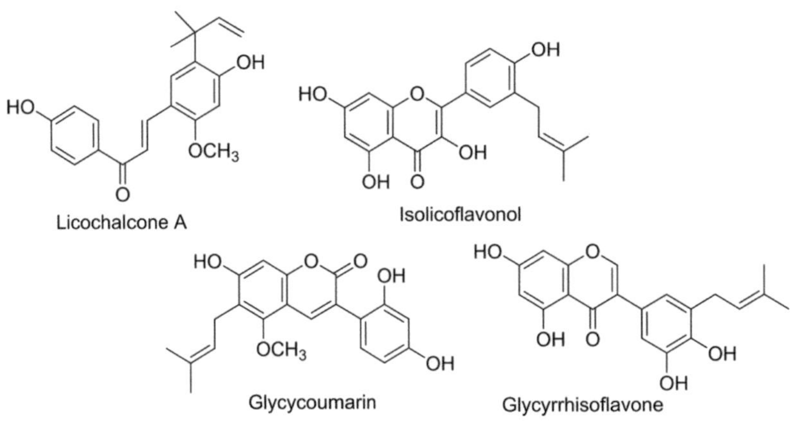

Figure 4. Licorice phenolics with anti-HIV effects.

http://dx.doi.org/10.5772/66419

2.3.3. *Effects on drug-resistant bacteria*

2.3.3.1. *Polyphenols are effective against methicillin-resistant Staphylococcus aureus*

Based on these studies, we pursued structural studies of licorice phenolics and also investigated the effectiveness of the licorice phenolics on drug-resistant bacteria. Surveillance under the Ministry of Health, Labour and Welfare within the Japanese government indicated that ca. 18,000 cases caused by methicillin-resistant *Staphylococcus aureus* (MRSA) in 2014 was reported for about 480 designated hospitals in Japan [33]. Since there are limited antibiotics and drugs (e.g., vancomycin and linezolid) available for the infectious diseases caused by MRSA, developing new candidates as remedies is essential. Indeed, hydrolyzable tannins such as tellimagrandin I and corilagin (in addition to an astringent constituent (-)-epicatechin gallate in green tea leaves) reportedly suppress the oxacillin resistance of MRSA strains. Therefore, we investigated licorice phenolics as candidates for new types of antibacterial drugs. Because acute toxicity is well understood for natural drug materials used in traditional medicine, low toxicity of their constituents is expected with some exceptions. Licorice has been widely used in traditional medicine, and its adverse effects (called pseudohyperaldosteronism) are ascribed to its main constituent glycyrrhizin. As such, its phenolic constituents could be candidates for developing novel remedies.

We examined the antibacterial effects of the phenolics isolated from licorice on four clinical isolates of MRSA (OM 481, OM505, OM 584, and OM 623) in addition to those of *Escherichia coli* and *Pseudomonas aeruginosa*. Although all of the examined phenolics did not show antibacterial effects on *E. coli* and *P. aeruginosa*, several compounds showed potent or moderate antibacterial effects on MRSA as shown below [15]. The compounds with a minimum inhibitory concentration (MIC) ≤ 32 μg/mL for the four MRSA strains are shown in **Table 2**. The following relationships were observed for both the structures and the antibacterial properties

Subgroups	Compound names (MIC)	Substituents
Chalcones	Licochalcone A (16 μg/mL)	α,α-Dimethylallyl × 1, OH × 2
Isoflavones	8-(γ,γ-Dimethylallyl)-wighteone (8 μg/mL)	Prenyl × 2, OH × 3
	Gancaonin G (16 μg/mL)	Prenyl × 1, OH × 2
	Isowighteone (32 μg/mL)	Prenyl × 1, OH × 2
	Isoangustone A (16 μg/mL)	Prenyl × 2, OH × 4
Isoflavanones	3′-(γ,γ-Dimethylallyl)-kievitone (8 μg/mL)	Prenyl × 2, OH × 4
	Licoisoflavanone (32 μg/mL)	Dimethylpyran × 1, OH × 3
Isoflavans	Glabridin (16 μg/mL)	Dimethylpyran × 1, OH × 2
	Glyasperin C (16 μg/mL)	Prenyl × 1, OH × 3
	Glyasperin D (16 μg/mL)	Prenyl × 1, OH × 2
	Licoricidin (16 μg/mL)	Prenyl × 2, OH × 3
3-Arylcoumarins	Glycycoumarin (16 μg/mL)	Prenyl × 1, OH × 3
	Licoarylcoumarin (32 μg/mL)	α,α-Dimethylallyl × 1, OH × 3
2-Arylbenzofurans	Licocoumarone (16 μg/mL)	Prenyl × 1, OH × 3
Benzyl phenyl ketones	Glicophenone (32 μg/mL)	Prenyl × 1, OH × 4
	Licoriphenone (16–32 μg/mL)	Prenyl × 1, OH × 3

Table 2. Licorice phenolics effective on MRSA strains.

of these compounds. All of these compounds had two or more phenolic hydroxyl groups and at least one prenyl (γ,γ-dimethylallyl) or equivalent (α,α-dimethylallyl or dimethylpyran) group. Comparisons of the anti-MRSA properties of the chalcones examined indicated the importance of a prenyl (or equivalent) group such as licochalcone A (MIC 16 μg/mL) > echinatin (MIC 64 or 128 μg/mL), licochalcone B (MIC 128 μg/mL), liquiritigenin (MIC 128 μg/mL), and tetrahydroxymethoxychalcone (MIC >128 μg/mL). Indeed, isoflavones with two prenyl groups (8-(γ,γ-dimethylallyl)-wighteone [MIC 8 μg/mL] and isoangustone A [MIC 16 μg/mL]) showed more potent anti-MRSA effects than those with one prenyl group (isowighteone [MIC 32 μg/mL], glycyrrhisoflavone [MIC 32 or 64 μg/mL], and glisoflavone [MIC 64 μg/mL]). Together with 8-(γ,γ-dimethylallyl)-wighteone, an isoflavanone with two prenyl groups, 3′-(γ,γ-dimethylallyl)-kievitone had the most potent anti-MRSA effects (MIC 8 μg/mL) among the examined compounds (**Figure 5**). Similarly, isoflavans with prenyl or equivalent group(s) (i.e., glyasperins C and D, glabridin, and licoricidin) showed more potent anti-MRSA effects (MIC 16 μg/mL) than those without a prenyl group ((3*R*)-vestitol [MIC 128 μg/mL]). The role of the prenyl group was tied to its affinity for the bacterial cell membranes. On the other hand, methylation of phenolic hydroxyl (OH) groups on the same structural skeleton weakened the anti-MRSA properties: glycycoumarin (MIC 16 μg/mL) (1 × OMe) > glycyrin (MIC 128 μg/mL) (2 × OMe) > glycyrin permethyl ether (MIC >128 μg/mL) (4 × OMe). Comparing the MIC of glycycoumarin with that of the corresponding coumestan, glycyrol [MIC >128 μg/mL] suggested that skeleton flexibility is also a factor impacting the anti-MRSA effects.

We further examined the suppressive effects of licorice phenolics with relatively potent anti-MRSA effects on the oxacillin resistance of the MRSA strains [15]. We compared MICs of oxacillin on MRSA strains with and without phenolics at half the MIC concentration or lower. For example, the addition of 16 μg/mL isowighteone (MIC 32 μg/mL) decreased oxacillin MIC to 1/8–1/4 of those without the addition (e.g., from 512 to 64 μg/mL and from 64 to 16 μg/mL) for the four MRSA strains (**Figure 6**). Similarly, the addition of 8 μg/mL of isoangustone A (MIC 16 μg/mL) decreased oxacillin MICs to 1/4–1/2, and the addition of 16 μg/mL of glicophenone (MIC 32 μg/mL) decreased oxacillin MIC to 1/8–1/2. Most notably, the addition of 8 μg/mL of licoricidin caused a decrease of oxacillin MIC to lower than

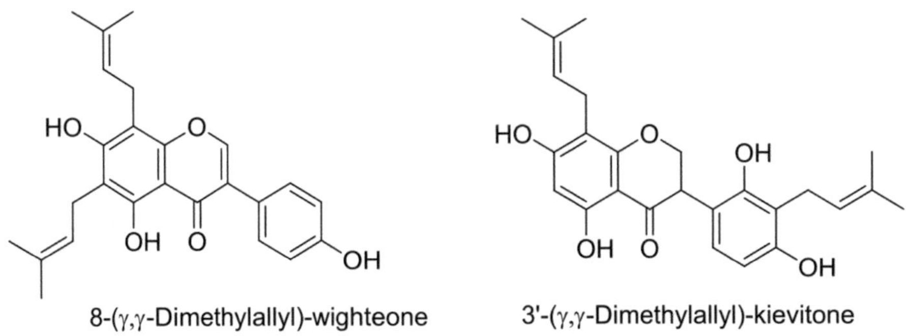

Figure 5. Licorice phenolics with the most potent antibacterial effect on MRSA.

http://dx.doi.org/10.5772/66419

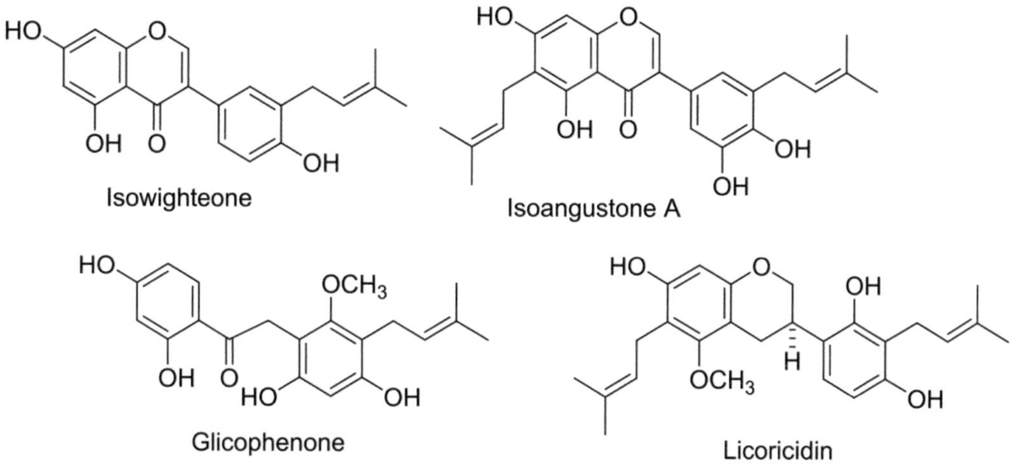

Figure 6. Licorice phenolics with suppressing effects on oxacillin resistance of MRSA.

0.5 μg/mL (lower than 1/1024–1/8). Even the addition of 4 μg/mL licoricidin decreased oxacillin MIC to 1/32–1/8 of those without the addition. Five of the other 6 phenolics, licochalcone A, licochalcone B, glicoricone, glisoflavone, and 3′-(γ,γ-dimethylallyl)-kievitone, also showed an analogous decreasing effect on at least two of the four MRSA strains. We also examined the effects of the combination of oxacillin (10 μg/mL) and licoricidin (8 μg/mL) on the bacterial growth of MRSA OM481, and the combination showed a bacteriostatic effect but not a bactericidal one. We also conducted a mechanistic study on the suppressive effects of the oxacillin resistance. The oxacillin resistance of MRSA OM481 has been attributed to the formation of a kind of protein-binding protein (PBP), PBP-2a (PBP-2′), instead of PBP-2. However, this formation in MRSA OM481 was not suppressed by the presence of licoricidin. Therefore, the suppression of the enzymatic function of PBP-2a or the binding to another PBP was attributed to the mechanism. On the other hand, the affinity of the lipophilic prenyl group to cell membranes was also supposed to be included in the mechanism, because all of the effective compounds have at least one prenyl (or equivalent) group.

Since the licorice phenolics with prenyl or equivalent substituents showed potent antibacterial effects on MRSA, we further investigated on the natural products with analogous structures contained in the fruits of *Psoralea corylifolia*, which have been known to have phenolic constituents with prenyl or related groups [34]. The following constituents of *P. corylifolia* showed MIC < 32 μg/mL for two MRSA strains, OM481 and OM584 (**Table 3**).

As shown above, the major constituent of the source material bakuchiol (meroterpene) together with isobavachalcone and corylifol B (chalcones) showed the most potent antibacterial effects among the constituents examined (**Figure 7**). We confirmed the importance of the presence of a prenyl or related lipophilic group in the molecules, suggesting that the participation of those groups is key within the bacterial membrane. Further mechanistic studies as shown by Refs. [35, 36] are expected.

Subgroups	Compound names (MIC)	Substituents
Flavones	Corylifol C (16 μg/mL)	Prenyl × 1, OH × 3
Flavanones	Bavachin (32 μg/mL)	Prenyl × 1, OH × 2
Isoflavones	Neobavaisoflavone (16 μg/mL)	Prenyl × 1, OH × 2
Chalcones	Corylifol B (8–16 μg/mL)	Prenyl × 1, OH × 4
	Isobavachalcone (8 μg/mL)	Prenyl × 1, OH × 3
Meroterpenes	Bakuchiol (8 μg/mL)	Ethenyldimethyloctadienyl × 1, OH × 1

Table 3. Phenolics from *Psoralea corylifolia* fruits effective on MRSA.

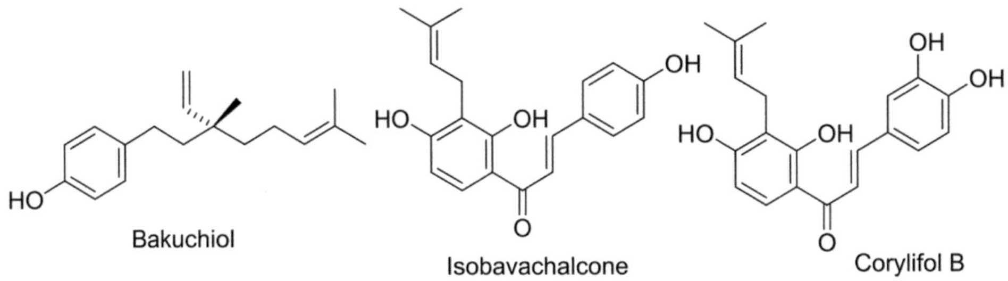

Figure 7. Phenolics with potent antibacterial effects on MRSA isolated from *Psoralea corylifolia* fruits.

Subgroups	Compounds (MIC)	Substituents
Isoflavones	8-(γ,γ-Dimethylallyl)-wighteone (8–16 μg/mL)	Prenyl × 2, OH × 3
	Glycyrrhisoflavone (32 μg/mL)	Prenyl × 1, OH × 4
	Isoangustone A (16 μg/mL)	Prenyl × 2, OH × 4
	7-*O*-Methylluteone (32 μg/mL)	Prenyl × 1, OH × 3
	Semilicoisoflavone B (32–64 μg/mL)	Dimethylpyran × 1, OH × 3
Isoflavans	Glyasperin C (16 μg/mL)	Prenyl × 1, OH × 3
	Glyasperin D (32–64 μg/mL)	Prenyl × 1, OH × 2
	Licoricidin (8 μg/mL)	Prenyl × 2, OH × 3
Isoflavanones	3′-(γ,γ-Dimethylallyl)-kievitone (16 μg/mL)	Prenyl × 2, OH × 4
	Glyasperin J (32 μg/mL)	Dimethylpyran × 1, prenyl × 1, OH × 3
3-Arylcoumarins	Glycycoumarin (16 μg/mL)	Prenyl × 1, OH × 3
	Glycyrin (16–32 μg/mL)	Prenyl × 1, OH × 2
	Licoarylcoumarin (16 μg/mL)	α,α-Dimethylallyl × 1, OH × 3
Coumestans	Isoglycerol (32–64 μg/mL)	Dimethyldihydropyran × 1, OH × 1
Pterocarpans	Demethylhomopterocarpan (32 μg/mL)	OH × 1
2-Arylbenzofurans	Gancaonin I (8–16 μg/mL)	Prenyl × 1, OH × 2
	Glycybenzofuran (32 μg/mL)	Prenyl × 1, OH × 3
	Licocoumarone (32 μg/mL)	Prenyl × 1, OH × 3
	4′-*O*-Methylglycybenzofuran (32 μg/mL)	Prenyl × 1, OH × 2
	Neoglycybenzofuran (16 μg/mL)	Prenyl × 1, OH × 3

Table 4. Licorice phenolics effective against VRE.

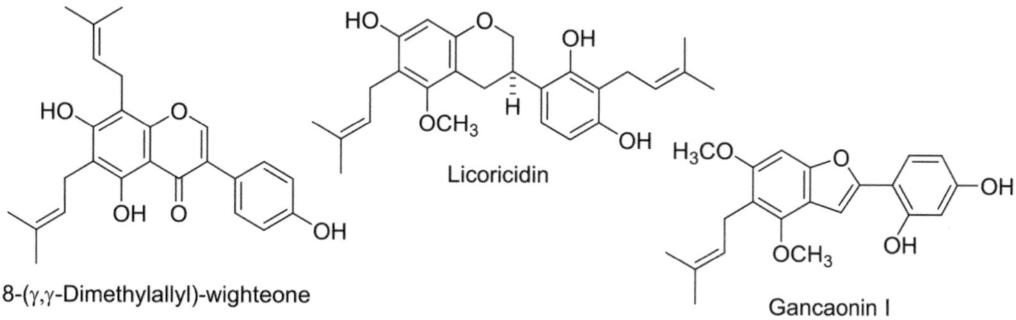

Figure 8. Licorice phenolics with potent antibacterial effects on VRE.

2.3.3.2. Polyphenols are effective against vancomycin-resistant Enterococci

We further examined the effects of phenolic constituents of licorice on vancomycin-resistant *Enterococcus* (VRE) species. Most antibiotics are ineffective against VRE, and only a few drugs such as linezolid or daptomycin can be used for VRE. Approximately 60–120 of the infected cases have been reported annually in Japan [37]; thus, infection of VRE in hospitals has become an important issue. Therefore, we have also investigated the plant constituents that are effective against VRE [38, 39].

The following strains of two species of VRE, *E. faecium* FN-1 and *E. faecalis* NCTC12201, were used for this study on licorice constituents. Various types of licorice phenolics showed antibacterial effects on these two VRE species, as shown below. The compounds that showed antibacterial effects on VRE with an MIC ≤ 32 μg/mL were classified into skeletons of the compounds (**Table 4**) [18, 19]. The following relationships were observed for the structures and the antibacterial properties of these compounds. All of the compounds have prenyl or equivalent groups and at least one hydroxyl group. The compound that showed the most potent effects on VRE was licoricidin (MIC 8 μg/mL), an isoflavan that has two prenyl and three hydroxyl groups. Comparisons of the isoflavans identified the following order of the antibacterial effects: licoricidin (with two prenyl groups) > glyasperins C and D (with one prenyl group). Comparisons of the compounds with the same isoflavone skeleton revealed that 8-(γ,γ-dimethylallyl)-wighteone and isoangustone A (both had two prenyl groups) showed more potent antibacterial effects on VRE (MIC 8–16 μg/mL) than glycyrrhisoflavone and 7-*O*-methylluteone (MIC 32 μg/mL) (both had one prenyl group). Among the 3-arylcoumarins, the coumestans, and the 2-arylbenzofurans, the compound with the most potent antibacterial effects is gancaonin I (MIC 8–16 μg/mL), with two hydroxyl groups and a prenyl group (**Figure 8**).

The contribution of hydroxyl groups seems to be less important in the cases of VRE than in the case of MRSA. For example, isoglycyrol and demethylhomopterocarpan both contained one hydroxyl group and showed moderate effects with MIC 32–64 μg/mL. Even for glyasperin J trimethyl ether, which has no hydroxyl groups, an MIC of 64 μg/mL was observed for both of the VRE species. On the other hand, 6,8-diprenylorobol with two prenyl groups and four hydroxyl groups showed weak effects (MIC 128 μg/mL). Therefore, respective structural factors or some balance of lipophilicity and hydrophilicity may contribute to the antibacterial effects, and this should be further investigated.

2.4. High-performance liquid chromatographic analysis of licorice phenolics

HPLC analysis revealed the presence of characteristic constituents depending on the original plant species. The *Japanese Pharmacopoeia* indicates that licorice used as a medicinal material must be derived from the origins of *G. uralensis* and *G. glabra*. Our analytical investigation on licorice materials from various sources indicated that the HPLC profiles could be separated into the following three types depending on several major constituents [21].

Type A: Using HPLC analysis, the standard materials established as *G. uralensis* in China were found to contain three relevant compounds: glycycoumarin, licopyranocoumarin, and licocoumarone (**Figure 9**). Conversely, HPLC analysis of the standard materials of *G. glabra* and *G. inflata* did not indicate the presence of these three compounds. All of the materials obtained from Japanese markets contained glycycoumarin, licopyranocoumarin, and licocoumarone, and several materials from Chinese markets also showed analogous HPLC patterns.

Type B: Analogously, the standard materials from *G. glabra* identified in China contained glabridin and glabrene (**Figure 10**), whereas these two were not observed for the standard materials from *G. uralensis* and *G. inflata*. The materials from Russia and Afghanistan revealed these two constituents, which were absent in the Japanese and Chinese market products.

Type C: The standard materials from *G. inflata* included licochalcones A and B (**Figure 11**), which were also present in some of the materials from Chinese markets.

These results suggest that glycycoumarin, licopyranocoumarin, and licocoumarone could be used as markers for *G. uralensis* (Type A). At the same time, glabridin and glabrene could be used as markers for *G. glabra* (Type B), and licochalcones A and B could be used as markers for *G. inflata* (Type C). However, licochalcone B was later isolated from a Japanese market sample.

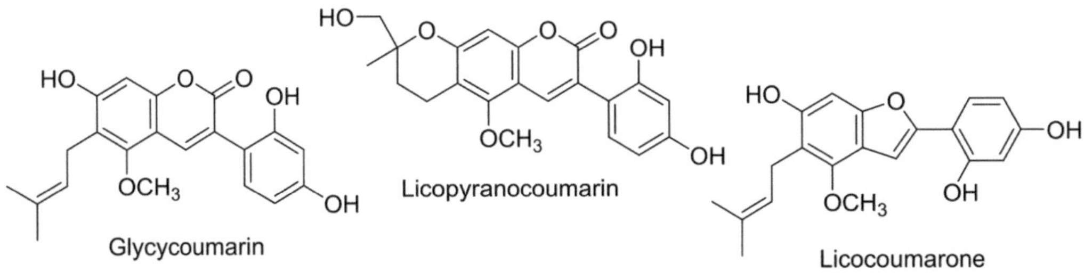

Figure 9. Characteristic phenolics observed in the extracts from *G. uralensis*.

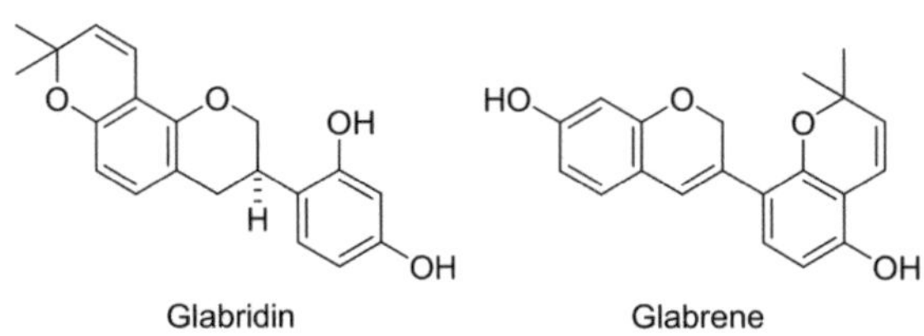

Figure 10. Characteristic phenolics observed in the extracts from *G. glabra*.

http://dx.doi.org/10.5772/66419

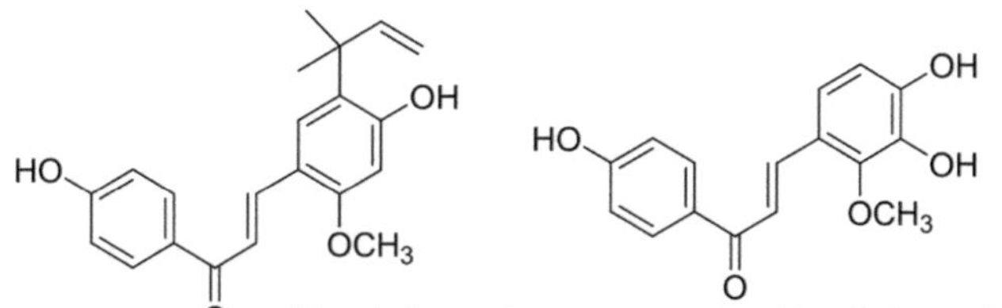

Figure 11. Characteristic phenolics observed in the extracts from *G. inflata*.

Furthermore, licoricidin, which was isolated from *G. uralensis* [15], has the same skeleton as glabridin. This finding suggests that glabridin might be a common constituent of *G. uralensis* and *G. glabra*, an assertion that is further strengthened by the fact that glabridin was recently found from *G. uralensis* [40]. Therefore, reinvestigation of marker compounds may be required, although glabrene and licochalcone A can be considered markers for *G. glabra* and *G. inflata*, respectively.

We performed HPLC analysis for the evaluation of crude drug materials to ascertain their pharmacological effects. The simultaneous HPLC analysis of eight major constituents of an extract from a material of a Japanese market was performed for evaluation as an anti-VRE material [19]. Using HPLC instruments combined with a photodiode-array detector (DAD) (LC-UV) or mass spectrometer (LC-MS) [19] would also effectively characterize such crude drug materials. Quantitative data and comparisons of the chromatographic patterns of representative licorice extracts, including unidentified HPLC peaks, are contributable to the evaluation of the materials. In addition, thin-layer chromatography (TLC) is a very useful method for visualizing phenolic constituents in plant extracts without special instruments [41], and development of high-performance (HP)TLC technique resulting in a better resolution of the constituent spots contributes largely in the analysis of plant constituents [42]. High-performance size-exclusion chromatography can be applied for estimating molecular sizes or molecular weight distribution of tannins [43] and also for estimating sizes of supermolecular complexes formed from polyphenols and proteins [26]. Gel electrophoresis is applicable for the analyses of polyphenol-protein complexes [44], too.

3. Conclusions

Licorice extracts contain various types of flavonoids and related compounds. In addition to the protein-binding properties and antioxidant effects, we examined their antiviral and antibacterial properties. The findings, especially those found in the studies of antibacterial phenolics in licorice using MRSA and VRE, emphasize the importance of lipophilic prenyl groups together with phenolic hydroxyl groups, in addition to the flexibility of their structural skeletons. Additional studies on these plant constituents are currently in progress [45]. Because naturally occurring polyphenols have structural limitations based on the biogenetic capability of plants, further studies with the aid of synthetic chemistry are expected for clarifying quantitative structure-activity relationship concerning their pharmacological effects and for optimizing candidates of new drugs.

4. Notes

The author (TH) regrets that the following errors were found: (1) The concentration 1 μg/mL of oxacillin in the figure legend on the effects of the combination of oxacillin and licoricidin from **Figure 2** in Ref. [15] should read 10 μg/mL as shown in the text of Ref. [15]; (2) the methoxyl and the hydroxyl groups in the structure of glycyrol in Refs. [18, 19] should be at C1 and C3, respectively, as shown in Ref. [34], and the structure of glycycoumarin in the Refs. [18] and [19] should be fixed as shown in Refs. [9, 15]; (3) the subgroup name 2-aryl-3-methylbenzofuran for gancaonin I in Ref. [19] is incorrect. Because gancaonin I does not have a methyl group on C3, it is classified in a subgroup of 2-arylbenzofuran as shown in **Table 4** in this chapter; (4) the name "reduced form of nicotinamide adenine dinucleotide phosphate (NADPH)" in Ref. [30] is an error and should read "NADH."

Author details

Tsutomu Hatano[1]*, Eerdunbayaer[1, 2], Yanmei Cui[1], Teruo Kuroda[3] and Yuuki Shimozu[1]

*Address all correspondence to: hatano-t@cc.okayama-u.ac.jp

1 Department of Natural Product Chemistry, Graduate School of Medicine, Dentistry and Pharmaceutical Sciences, Okayama University, Okayama, Japan

2 Chenguang Biotech Group, Co., Ltd., Quzhou County, Hebei Province, China

3 Department of Microbiology, Graduate School of Biomedical & Health Sciences, Hiroshima University, Hiroshima, Japan

References

[1] Shibata S (2000) A drug over the millennia: Pharmacognosy, chemistry, and pharmacology of licorice. Yakugaku Zasshi, 120, 849–862.

[2] Shibata S, Saitoh T (1978) Flavonoid compounds in licorice root. J. Indian Chem. Soc., 55, 1184–1191.

[3] Nomura T, Fukai T (1998) Phenolic constituents of licorice (*Glycyrrhiza* species). Fortschr. Chem. Org. Naturst., 73, 1–140.

[4] Mitscher LA, Park YH, Clark D, Beal JL (1980) Antimicrobial agents from higher plants. Antimicrobial isoflavanoids and related substances from *Glycyrrhiza glabra* L. var. *typica*. J. Nat. Prod., 43, 259–269.

[5] Demizu S, Kajiyama K, Takahashi K, Hiraga Y, Yamamoto S, Tamura Y, Okada K, Kinoshita T (1988) Antioxidant and antimicrobial constituents of licorice: Isolation and structure elucidation of a new benzofuran derivative. Chem. Pharm. Bull., 36, 3474–3479.

[6] Okuda T, Yoshida T, Hatano T (1992) Pharmacologically active tannins isolated from medicinal plants. Basic Life Sci., 59, 539–569.

[7] Yoshida T, Hatano T, Ito H (2000) Chemistry and function of vegetable polyphenols with high molecular weights. Biofactors, 13, 121–125.

[8] Quideau S (ed.) (2009) Chemistry and biology of ellagitannins, an underestimated class of bioactive plant polyphenols. World Scientific Publishing, Singapore.

[9] Hatano T, Kagawa H, Yasuhara T, Okuda T (1988) Two new flavonoids and other constituents in licorice root: Their relative astringency and radical scavenging effects. Chem. Pharm. Bull., 36, 2090–2097.

[10] Okuda T, Yoshida T, Hatano T (1988) Application of centrifugal partition chromatography to tannins and related polyphenols. J. Liq. Chromatogr., 11, 2447–2454.

[11] Hatano T, Yasuhara T, Miyamoto K, Okuda T (1988) Anti-human immunodeficiency virus phenolics from licorice. Chem. Pharm. Bull., 36, 2286–2288.

[12] Hatano T, Yasuhara T, Fukuda T, Noro T, Okuda T (1989) Phenolic constituents of licorice. II. Structures of licopyranocoumarin, licoarylcoumarin and glisoflavone, and inhibitory effects of licorice phenolics on xanthine oxidase. Chem. Pharm. Bull., 37, 3005–3009.

[13] Okuda T, Yoshida T, Hatano T, Mori K, Fukuda T (1990) Fractionation of pharmacologically active plant polyphenols by centrifugal partition chromatography. J. Liq. Chromatogr., 13, 3637–3650.

[14] Hatano T, Fukuda T, Miyase T, Noro T, Okuda T (1991) Phenolic constituents of licorice. III. Structures of glicoricone, licofuranone, and inhibitory effects of licorice constituents on monoamine oxidase. Chem. Pharm. Bull., 39, 1238–1243.

[15] Hatano T, Shintani Y, Aga Y, Shiota S, Tsuchiya T, Yoshida T (2000) Phenolic constituents of licorice. VIII. Structures of glicophenone and glicoisoflavanone, and effects of licorice phenolics on methicillin-resistant *Staphylococcus aureus*. Chem. Pharm. Bull., 48, 1286–1292.

[16] Hatano T, Aga Y, Shintani Y, Ito H, Okuda T, Yoshida T (2000) Minor flavonoids from licorice. Phytochemistry, 55, 959–963.

[17] Hatano T, Takagi M, Ito H, Yoshida T (1998) Acylated flavonoid glycosides and accompanying phenolics from licorice. Phytochemistry, 47, 287–293.

[18] Eerdunbayaer, Orabi MA, Aoyama H, Kuroda T, Hatano T (2014) Structures of two new flavonoids and effects of licorice phenolics on vancomycin-resistant *Enterococcus* species. Molecules, 19, 3883–3897.

[19] Eerdunbayaer, Orabi MA, Aoyama H, Kuroda T, Hatano T (2014) Structures of new phenolics isolated from licorice, and the effectiveness of licorice phenolics on vancomycin-resistant *Enterococci*. Molecules, 19, 13027–13041.

[20] Hatano T, Takagi M, Ito H, Yoshida T (1997) Phenolic constituents of liquorice. VII. A new chalcone with a potent radical-scavenging activity and accompanying phenolics from liquorice. Chem. Pharm. Bull., 45, 1485–1492.

[21] Hatano T, Fukuda T, Liu YZ, Noro T, Okuda T (1991) Phenolic constituents of licorice. IV. Correlation of phenolic constituents and licorice specimens from various sources, and inhibitory effects of licorice extracts on xanthine oxidase and monoamine oxidase. Yakugaku Zasshi, 111, 311–321 (in Japanese).

[22] Haslam E (1998) Practical polyphenolics: From structure to molecular recognition and physiological action. Cambridge University Press, Cambridge.

[23] Baxter NJ, Lilley TH, Haslam E, Williamson MP (1997) Multiple interactions between polyphenols and a salivary proline-rich protein repeat result in complexation and precipitation. Biochemistry, 36, 5566–5577.

[24] Richard T, Lefeuvre D, Descendit A, Quideau S, Monti JP (2006) Recognition characters in peptide-polyphenol complex formation. Biochim. Biophys. Acta, 1760, 951–958.

[25] Hatano T, Yoshida T, Hemingway RW (1999) Interaction of flavonoids with peptides and proteins and conformations of dimeric flavonoids in solution. In: Plant polyphenols 2: Chemistry, biology, pharmacology, ecology (Edited by Gross GG, Hemingway RW, Yoshida T), Kluwer Academic/Plenum Publishers, New York, pp. 509–526.

[26] Hatano T, Hori M, Hemingway RW, Yoshida T (2003) Size exclusion chromatographic analysis of polyphenol-serum albumin complexes. Phytochemistry, 63, 817–823.

[27] Nozaki A, Kimura T, Ito H, Hatano T (2009) Interaction of polyphenolic metabolites with human serum albumin: A circular dichroism study. Chem. Pharm. Bull., 57, 1019–1023.

[28] Okuda T, Mori K, Hatano T (1985) Relationship of the structures of tannins to the binding activities with hemoglobin and methylene blue. Chem. Pharm. Bull., 33, 1424–1433.

[29] Kimura Y, Okuda H, Okuda T, Arichi S (1988) Effects of chalcones isolated from licorice roots on leukotriene biosynthesis in human polymorphonuclear neutrophils. Phytotherapy Res., 2, 140–145.

[30] Hatano T, Yoshida T (1998) Bioactive phenolics from licorice: Their radical-scavenging effects, inhibitory effects on oxidative enzymes and antiviral effects. In: Towards natural medicine research in the twenty first century (Edited by Ageta H, Aimi N, Ebizuka Y, Fujita T, Honda G), Elsevier, Amsterdam, pp. 261–272.

[31] Nakashima H, Murakami T, Yamamoto N, Sakagami H, Tanuma S, Hatano T, Yoshida T, Okuda T (1992) Inhibition of human immunodeficiency viral replication by tannins and related compounds. Antiviral Res., 18, 91–103.

[32] Uchiumi F, Hatano T, Ito H, Yoshida T, Tanuma S (2003) Transcriptional suppression of the HIV promoter by natural compounds. Antiviral Res., 58, 89–98.

[33] http://www.nih.go.jp/niid/images/idwr/ydata/2014/Syuukei/Syu_11_1. xlsx (http://www.nih.go.jp/niid/ja/survei/2270-idwr/nenpou/6142-syulist2014.html)

[34] Cui Y, Taniguchi S, Kuroda T, Hatano T (2015) Constituents of *Psoralea corylifolia* fruits and their effects on methicillin-resistant *Staphylococcus aureus*. Molecules, 20, 12500–12511.

[35] Shiota S, Shimizu M, Sugiyama J, Morita Y, Mizushima T, Tsuchiya T (2004) Mechanisms of action of corilagin and tellimagrandin I that remarkably potentiate the activity of beta-lactams against methicillin-resistant *Staphylococcus aureus*. Microbiol. Immunol., 48, 67–73.

[36] Kusuda M, Inada K, Ogawa TO, Yoshida T, Shiota S, Tsuchiya T, Hatano T (2006) Polyphenolic constituent structures of *Zanthoxylum piperitum* fruit and the antibacterial effects of its polymeric procyanidin on methicillin-resistant *Staphylococcus aureus*. Biosci. Biotechnol. Biochem., 70, 1423–1431.

[37] http://idsc.nih.go.jp/idwr/ydata/report-Ja.html

[38] Horiuchi K, Shiota S, Hatano T, Yoshida T, Kuroda T, Tsuchiya T (2007) Antimicrobial activity of oleanolic acid from *Salvia officinalis* and related compounds on vancomycin-resistant enterococci (VRE). Biol. Pharm. Bull., 30, 1147–1149.

[39] Okamura S, Nishiyama E, Yamazaki T, Otsuka N, Taniguchi S, Ogawa W, Hatano T, Tsuchiya T, Kuroda T (2015) Action mechanism of 6, 6′-dihydroxythiobinupharidine from *Nuphar japonicum*, which showed anti-MRSA and anti-VRE activities. Biochim. Biophys. Acta, 1850, 1245–1252.

[40] Shirahata T, Terada T, Yoshimatsu K, Fuchino H, Kawano N, Inui T, Tamura K, Fukuda T, Kawahara N, Kobayashi N (2016) Preparation of standardized plots for evaluation of licorice using ^{1}H NMR metabolic profiling. Abstracts, 63th Annual Meeting of the Japanese Society of Pharmacognosy, Toyama, p. 238 (in Japanese).

[41] Wagner H, Bladt S (1996) Plant drug analysis, 2nd ed. Springer, Heidelberg.

[42] Cimpoiu C (2006) Analysis of some natural antioxidants by thin-layer chromatography and high performance thin-layer chromatography. J. Liq. Chromatogr. Relat. Tech., 29, 1125–1142.

[43] Kaufman RC, Tilley M, Bean SR, Tuinstra MR (2009) Improved characterization of sorghum tannins using size-exclusion chromatography. Cereal Chem., 86, 369–371.

[44] Kusuda M, Hatano T, Yoshida T (2006) Water-soluble complexes formed by natural polyphenols and bovine serum albumin: Evidence from gel electrophoresis. Biosci. Biotech. Biochem., 70, 152–160.

[45] Shimozu Y (2016) Polyphenols effective on drug resistant bacteria and the mechanisms. In: Polyphenols: New trends of studies and developments on functional constituents in plants (Edited by Hatano T, Shimoda H), CMC Publishing, Tokyo, pp. 65–72 (in Japanese).

Chapter 5

Phenolics from *Glycyrrhiza glabra* and *G. uralensis* Roots and Their PPAR-γ Ligand-Binding Activity: Possible Application for Amelioration of Type 2 Diabetes

Minpei Kuroda and Yoshihiro Mimaki

Additional information is available at the end of the chapter

http://dx.doi.org/10.5772/67406

Abstract

The EtOH extract of *Glycyrrhiza glabra* roots and the EtOAc extract of *Glycyrrhiza uralensis* roots exhibited considerable PPAR-γ ligand-binding activity. Bioassay-guided fractionation of these extracts resulted in the isolation of 52 phenolics, including 11 novel ones. The PPAR-γ ligand-binding activity of more than 10 isolated phenolics at 10 μg/mL was approximately three times greater than that of 0.5 μM triglitazone. Glycyrin (**44**), isolated from the EtOAc extract of *G. uralensis* roots as a PPAR-γ ligand, reduced the blood glucose levels of genetically diabetic KK-A^y mice through its PPAR-γ ligand-binding activity.

Keywords: phenolics, *Glycyrrhiza glabra, Glycyrrhiza uralensis*, PPAR-γ, metabolic syndrome

1. Introduction

Peroxisome proliferator-activated receptor (PPAR)-γ is the primary molecular target for insulin-sensitizing thiazolidinedione drugs. These drugs activate PPAR-γ, increasing the number of small adipocytes that differentiate from preadipocytes and inducing apoptosis in large adipocytes. Because small adipocytes function normally, whereas large adipocytes hyperproduce and hypersecrete adipocytokines, an increased ratio of small adipocytes to large adipocytes improves insulin resistance. Therefore, compounds with PPAR-γ ligand-binding activity may be useful for the prevention and improvement of type 2 diabetes, a representative insulin resistance syndrome. We found that the EtOH extract of *Glycyrrhiza glabra* roots and the EtOAc extract of *G. uralensis* roots exhibited higher activity than did the other materials tested. Bioassay-guided fractionation of these extracts resulted in the isolation of 52 phenolics, including 11 novel ones [1, 2].

In this chapter, we describe the results of the bioassay-guided fractionation of *G. glabra* and *G. uralensis* roots using a GAL-4-PPAR-γ chimera assay method.

2. PPAR-γ ligand-binding activity

PPAR-γ ligand-binding activity was assessed using a GAL-4-PPAR-γ chimera assay system (**Figure 1**) [3]. CV-1 monkey kidney cells from the American Type Culture Collection (ATCC) were suspended in Dulbecco's Modified Eagle medium (DMEM) containing 10% fetal bovine serum (FBS), 50 IU/mL Penicillin G sodium salt, 50 μg/mL streptomycin sulfate, and 37 mg/L ascorbic acid. The cells were then inoculated into a 96-well culture plate at 6×10^3 cells/well and incubated in 5% CO_2/air at 37°C for 24 h. Cells were washed with OPTI-minimum essential medium (MEM) and pM-hPPAR-γ and p4 × UASg-tk-luc were transfected into cells using LipofectAMINE PLUS (Gibco). pM and p4 × UASg-tk-luc were transfected into CV-1 cells as a mock control. Twenty-four hours after transfection, the medium was changed to DMEM containing 10% charcoal-treated FBS [4] and the cells were further cultured for 24 h. The cells were then washed with phosphate-buffered saline containing Ca^{2+} and Mg^{2+}, and luciferase activity was measured using LucLite (Perkin-Elmer). Luminescence intensity was measured using a TopCount Microplate scintillation/luminescence counter. PPAR-γ ligand-binding activity was expressed as the relative luminescence intensity (test group/control group) determined for each sample.

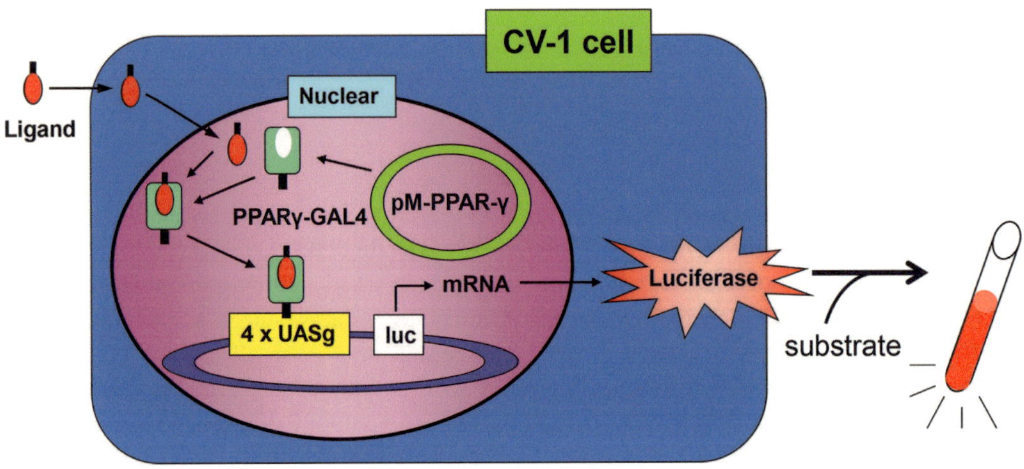

Figure 1. GAL4-PPAR-γ chimera assay system.

3. Isolation and structural determination of phenolic compounds from *G. glabra*

The roots of *G. glabra* (4.0 kg) were extracted twice with 20 L of 95% EtOH for 2 h at 45°C. The extracts were combined and concentrated under reduced pressure to give a 95% EtOH extract (120 g). The extract exhibited a relative luminescence intensity of 2.2 at a sample concentration of 5 μg/mL, indicating a PPAR-γ ligand-binding activity that was almost as strong as that of 0.5 μM troglitazone (TRG), a potent synthetic PPAR-γ agonist. The extract was chromatographed on a silica gel column eluted with $CHCl_3$-MeOH gradients (19:1; 9:1; 2:1) and finally with MeOH. After removal of solvent, the fraction eluted with $CHCl_3$-MeOH (19:1) yielded 85 g of material that showed notable PPAR-γ ligand-binding activity (**Figure 2**). A series of chromatographic separations were then performed, resulting in 10 new phenolic compounds [**1** (8.0 mg), **2** (13.8 mg), **3** (1.6 mg), **4** (6.9 mg), **5** (18.5 mg), **6** (8.6 mg), **7** (18.5 mg), **8** (4.9 mg), **9** (7.3 mg), **10** (30.2 mg)] (**Figure 3**). In addition, 29 known phenolic compounds were obtained and identified by comparison of physical and spectral data with those reported in the literature. The following known phenolic compounds were identified in the $CHCl_3$-MeOH (19:1) fraction: echinatin (**11**, 5.4 mg) [5], lichocalcone B (**12**, 17.3 mg) [6], morachalcone A (**13**, 14.1 mg) [7], 2′,3,4′-trihydroxy-3′-γ,γ-dimethylallyl-6″,6″-dimethylpyrano[2″,3″:4,5]chalcone (**14**, 17.4 mg) [8], 1-(2′,4′-dihydroxyphenyl)-2-hydroxy-3-(4″-hydroxyphenyl)-1-propanone (**15**, 5.8 mg) [9], kanzonol Y (**16**, 2.5 mg) [10], (3*R*)-vestitol (**17**, 10.5 mg) [11], (3*R*)-2′,3′,7-trihydroxy-4′-methoxyisoflavan (**18**, 8.1 mg) [12], kanzonol X (**19**, 37.1 mg) [10], glabridin (**20**, 193 mg) [13], 4′-*O*-methylglabridin (**21**, 11.4 mg) [14], 3′-hydroxy-4′-*O*-methylglabridin (**22**, 54.7 mg) [15],

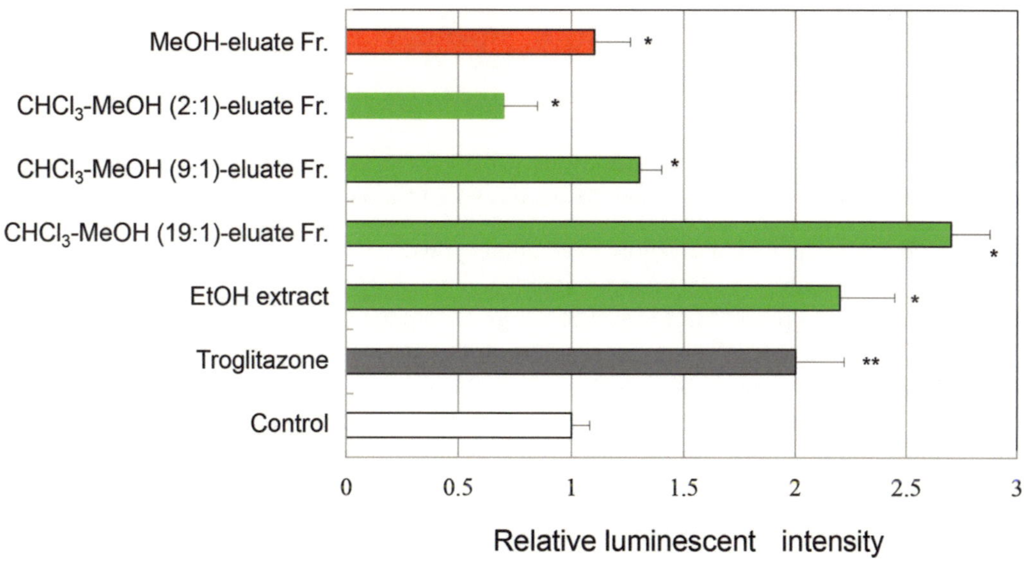

Figure 2. PPAR-γ ligand-binding activity of *G. glabra* extract and fractions [1]. PPAR-γ ligand-binding activity of the extract and fractions (5 μg/mL), as well as that of troglitazone (0.5 μM) used as a positive control, was measured using a GAL-4-PPAR-γ chimera assay. Statistical significance is indicated as * ($p < 0.05$) or ** ($p < 0.01$) as determined by Dunnett's multiple comparison test.

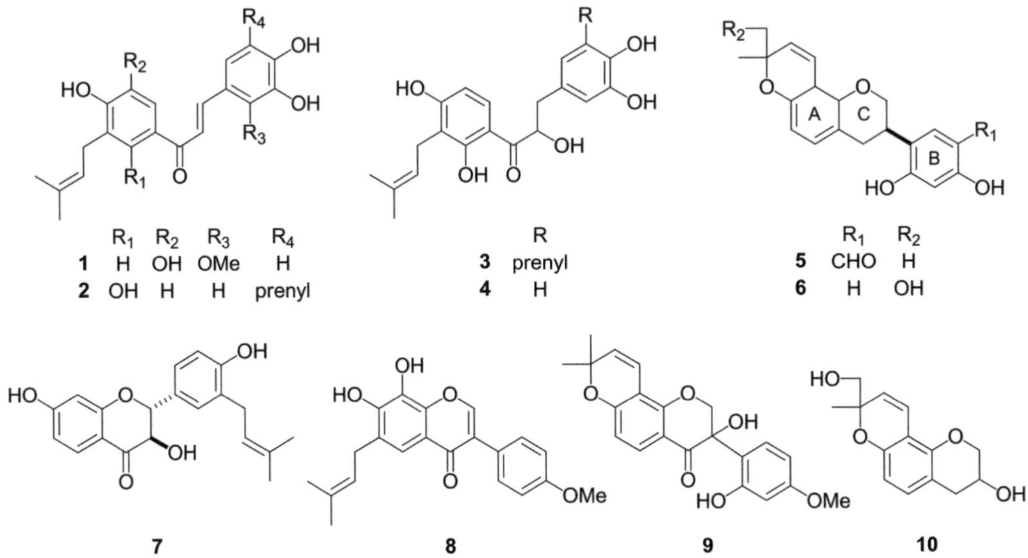

Figure 3. Structures of **1–10** isolated from *G. glabra* roots [1].

hispaglabridin A (**23**, 13.7 mg) [14], hispaglabridin B (**24**, 10.7 mg) [14], glabrene (**25**, 28.8 mg) [16], kanzonol W (**26**, 3.0 mg) [10], glabrocoumarin (**27**, 16.4 mg) [17], shinpterocarpin (**28**, 41.0 mg) [18], *O*-methylshinpterocarpin (**29**, 32.4 mg) [18], licoagrocarpin (**30**, 6.1 mg) [19], licoflavanone A (**31**, 4.8 mg) [20], glabrol (**32**, 13.5 mg) [13], shinflavanone (**33**, 7.8 mg) [18], euchrenone a5 (**34**, 1.5 mg) [21], xambioona (**35**, 8.0 mg) [22], gancaonin L (**36**, 8.8 mg) [23], glabrone (**37**, 15.5 mg) [24], kanzonol U (**38**, 21.6 mg) [11], and 8,8-dimethyl-3,4-dihydro-2*H*,8*H*-pyrano[2,3-*f*]-chromon-3-ol (**39**, 17.4 mg) [25] (**Figure 4**). The structures of isolated compounds were classified into 12 groups: chalcones (**1–4**, **11–16**), isoflavans (**5**, **6**, **17–24**), an isoflavone (**25**), 3-arylcoumarins (**26**, **27**), pterocarpans (**28–30**), a flavone (**31**), a flavanol (**7**), flavanones (**32–35**), isoflavones (**8**, **36**, **37**), an isoflavane (**9**), an 2-aryl benzofuran (**38**), and chromones (**10**, **39**). Compounds **13**, **15**, **17**, **18**, and **36** were isolated from *G. glabra* for the first time.

Compound **1** was isolated as a yellow amorphous powder with a formula of $C_{21}H_{22}O_6$ determined by high-resolution electrospray ionization mass spectrometry (HRESIMS), which showed an accurate $[M+H]^+$ ion at *m*/*z* 371.1487. Compound **1** had an absorption maxima at 366 and 248 nm in its UV spectrum and absorbance bands at 3427 cm^{-1} (hydroxy groups), 1625 cm^{-1} (conjugated carbonyl group), and 1595, 1507, and 1469 cm^{-1} (aromatic rings) in its IR spectrum. The ^1H NMR spectrum of **1** (acetone-d_6) contained signals for two *trans*-coupled protons at δ_H 7.91 and 7.67 (each d, *J* = 15.7 Hz), *ortho*-coupled aromatic protons at δ_H 7.25 and 6.72 (each d, *J* = 8.5 Hz), *meta*-coupled aromatic protons at δ_H 7.55 and 7.51 (each d, *J* = 1.9 Hz), and methoxy protons at δ_H 3.88 (s). In addition, the ^1H NMR spectrum indicated the presence of a prenyl (3-methyl-2-butenyl) group [δ_H 5.40 (1H, m), 3.43 (2H, br d, *J* = 7.3 Hz), 1.77 and 1.75 (each 3H, br s)]. These data suggested that **1** was a chalcone derivative with four hydroxy groups, a methoxy group, and a prenyl group. Long-range correlations were observed in the heteronuclear multiple bond coherence (HMBC) spectrum of **1** (**Figure 5**) between H-2 (δ_H 7.51) and C═O (carbonyl, δ_C 188.0)/C-3 (δ_C 144.6)/C-4 (δ_C 148.3)

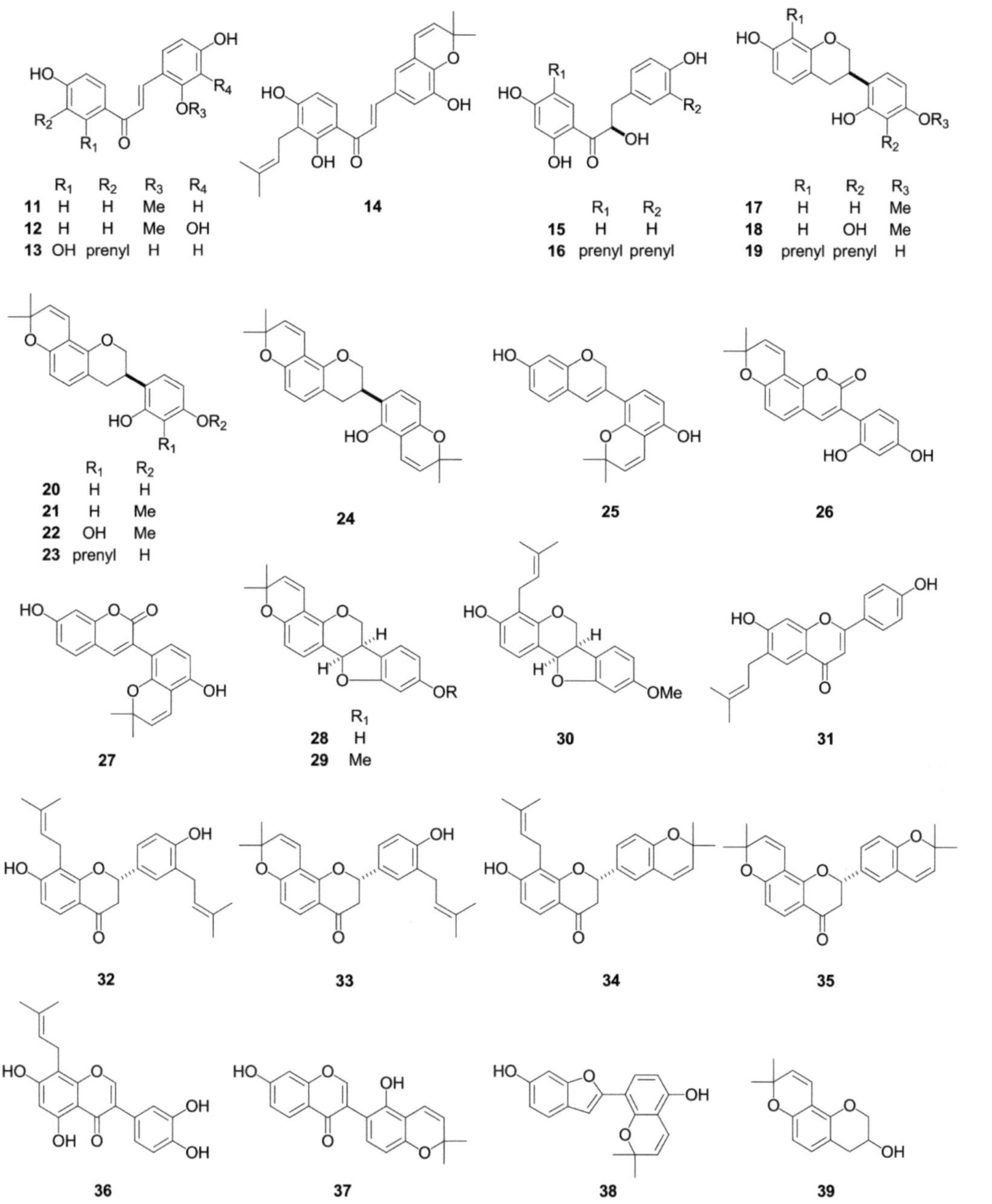

Figure 4. Structures of **11–39** isolated from *G. glabra* roots [1].

and between H-6 (δ_H 7.55) and C=O/C-1 (δ_C 130.7), indicating that two hydroxy groups were attached to C-3 and C-4. HMBC correlations between H-1″ (δ_H 3.43) and C-4/C-6 (δ_C 122.8) and between H-2″ (δ_H 5.40) and C-5 (δ_C 128.2) indicated the existence of a prenyl group at C-5. The structure of the B-ring moiety attributed to 3′,4′-dihydroxy-2′-methoxyphenyl and its linkage to C-β of the *trans*-olefinic group were determined by HMBC correlations between

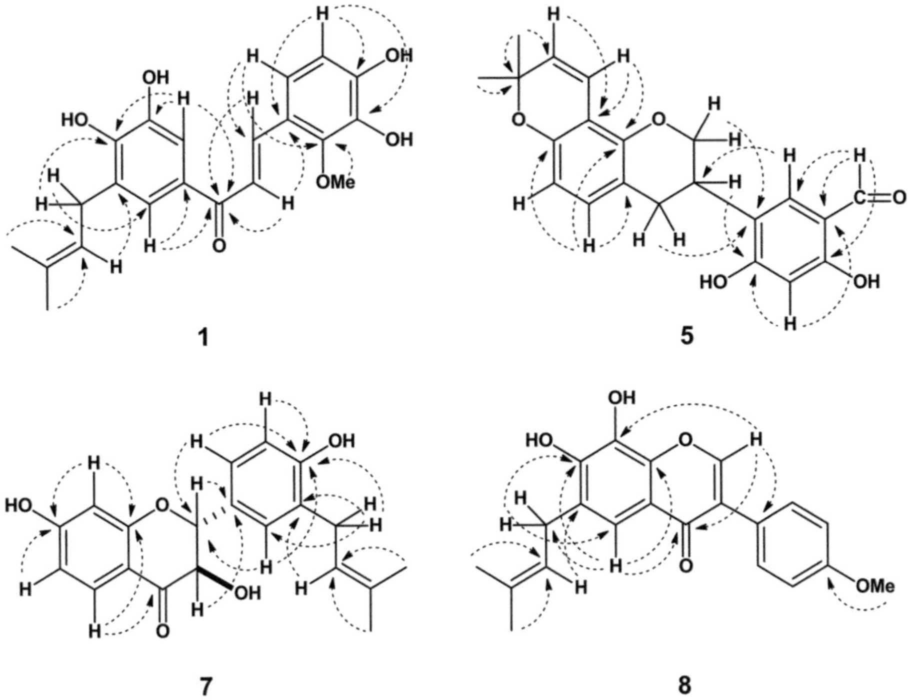

Figure 5. Key HMBC correlations of **1**, **5**, **7**, and **8** [1].

H-5′ (δ_H 6.72) and C-1′ (δ_C 121.0)/C-3′ (δ_C 138.7)/C-4′ (δ_C 149.0), H-6′ (δ_H 7.25) and C-β (δ_C 138.4)/C-2′ (δ_C 148.7), and methoxy protons and C-2′. Therefore, the structure of **1** was assigned as 3,3′,4,4′-tetrahydroxy-2′-methoxy-5-prenylchalcone.

Compound **5** was isolated as a yellow amorphous powder with a molecular formula of $C_{21}H_{20}O_5$ determined by HRESIMS. The ^{1}H NMR spectrum of **5** indicated signals characteristic of an isoflavan skeleton at δ_H 4.43 (ddd, *J* = 10.2, 3.4, 2.2 Hz, H-2a), 4.07 (dd, *J* = 10.2, 10.2 Hz, H-2b), 3.54 (m, H-3), 3.07 (dd, *J* = 15.5, 11.1 Hz, H-4a), and 2.90 (ddd, *J* = 15.5, 5.0, 2.2 Hz, H-4b). In addition, the spectrum of **5** indicated signals that we assigned to two aromatic protons at δ_H 7.58 and 6.49 (each s), *ortho*-coupled aromatic protons at δ_H 6.87 and 6.32 (each d, *J* = 8.2 Hz), and a 2,2-dimethylpyran ring at δ_H 6.63 and 5.65 (each 1H, d, *J* = 9.8 Hz) and δ_H 1.40 and 1.38 (each 3H, s). Compound **5** and glabridin (**20**) have similar features in their ^{1}H NMR spectra. Moreover, the ^{1}H and ^{13}C NMR signals at δ_H 9.77 and δ_C 195.3 indicated the presence of a formyl group, which was attached at C-5′, as determined by the HMBC correlations between the formyl proton signal and C-4′ (δ_C 163.6)/C-5′ (δ_C 115.4)/C-6′ (δ_C 133.9) (**Figure 5**). The circular dichroism (CD) profile of **5** was the same as that of synthetic 5′-formylglabridin prepared by formylation of **20**, indicating that the absolute configuration at C-3 was *R*. Therefore, the structure of **5** was assigned as 5′-formyl glabridin. It was notable that **5** was the first naturally occurring isoflavan with a formyl group in the B-ring portion of the compound.

Compound **7** was isolated as a yellow powder with a molecular formula of $C_{20}H_{20}O_5$ determined by HRESIMS. Compound **7** had an absorption maxima at 313 and 276 nm in its UV spectrum and absorption bands at 3374 cm^{-1} (hydroxy groups), 1673 cm^{-1} (a carbonyl group), and 1608, 1502, and 1463 cm^{-1} (aromatic rings) in its IR spectrum. The ^1H NMR spectrum of **7** showed signals that we assigned to a prenyl group at δ_H 5.39 (1H, m), 3.38 (2H, d, *J* = 7.3 Hz), and 1.74 and 1.72 (each 3H, br s), and two methines bearing an oxygen function at δ_H 5.03 and 4.59 (each d, *J* = 11.9 Hz). Furthermore, two 1,3,4-trisubstituted aromatic rings were identified from six aromatic protons comprising two ABX-type spin-coupling systems at δ_H 7.74 (d, *J* = 8.6 Hz), 6.64 (dd, *J* = 8.6, 2.2 Hz), and 6.41 (d, *J* = 2.2 Hz) and δ_H 7.35 (d, *J* = 2.0 Hz), 7.27 (dd, *J* = 8.2, 2.0 Hz), and 6.90 (d, *J* = 8.2 Hz). The above data indicated that **7** was a dihydroxyflavan-3-ol derivative with a prenyl unit. The HMBC correlations between H-5 (δ_H 7.74) and C-4 (δ_C 192.7)/C-9 (δ_C 164.1), H-8 (δ_H 6.41) and C-7 (δ_C 165.4)/C-9, H-6 (δ_H 6.64) and C-7, H-2′ (δ_H 7.35) and C-2 (δ_C 84.6)/C-4′ (δ_C 155.8), H-6′ (δ_H 7.27) and C-2/C-4′, and H-1″ (δ_H 3.38) and C-2′ (δ_C 130.0)/C-3′ (δ_C 128.1)/C-4′ indicated that two hydroxy groups and a prenyl group were attached to C-7, C-4′, and C-3′, respectively (**Figure 5**). In the CD spectrum of **7**, the positive Cotton effects at 210, 240, and 334 nm and the negative Cotton effect at 304 nm indicated absolute configurations of 2*R* and 3*R* [26]. Therefore, the structure of **7** was identified as (2*R*,3*R*)-3,4′,7-trihydroxy-3′-prenylflavanone.

The following suggested that compound **8** ($C_{21}H_{20}O_5$) was an isoflavone derivative: a UV absorption maximum at λ_{max} 263 nm [27], a proton resonance at δ_H 8.16 (1H, s), and a corresponding oxygen-bearing olefinic carbon signal at δ_C 152.2. The ^1H NMR spectrum of **8** contained signals for an aromatic proton at δ_H 7.54 (s), *p*-disubstituted aromatic protons at δ_H 7.55 and 6.98 (each d, *J* = 8.8 Hz), and methoxy protons at δ 3.84 (3H, s). In addition, the ^1H NMR spectrum implied the presence of a prenyl unit [δ_H 5.41 (1H, m), 3.56 (2H, d, *J* = 7.3 Hz), and 1.76 (3H × 2, br s)]. In the HMBC spectrum of **8** (**Figure 5**), correlation peaks were observed between H-5 (δ_H 7.54) and C-4 (δ_C 175.4)/C-7 (δ_C 148.7)/C-9 (δ_C 145.7)/C-1″ (δ_C 28.4), methoxy protons (δ_H 3.84) and C-4′ (δ_C 159.9), and H-2 (δ_H 8.16) and C-8 (δ_C 145.7), indicating that two hydroxy groups were attached to C-7 and C-8, a methoxy group to C-4′, and a prenyl group to C-6. Therefore, the structure of **8** was found to be 7,8-dihydroxy-4′-methoxy-6-prenylisoflavanone.

In the same way, the structures of **2–4**, **6**, **9**, and **10** were established as shown in **Figure 3**. Compounds **3**, **4**, and **9** showed neither specific rotation nor Cotton effects in their CD spectra, indicating that these compounds were racemates.

4. PPAR-γ ligand-binding activity of compounds 1–39 isolated from *G. glabra*

Compounds **5**, **7**, **11**, **18**, **19**, **26**, **28**, **31–33**, **36**, and **37** showed significant PPAR-γ ligand-binding activity. Among these compounds, the prenylflavone derivative licoflavanone A (**31**) was the most potent (**Figure 6**). These active compounds likely contributed the most to the PPAR-γ ligand-binding activity of the EtOH extract. The isoflavone derivative, kanzonol X (**19**), and flavanone derivative, glabrol (**32**), both had two prenyl units and exhibited potent ligand-binding activity. Hispaglabridin B (**24**) and xambioona (**35**), in which two prenyl units were cyclized to form two six-membered rings, exhibited weaker ligand-binding activities than **19** and **32** did, suggesting

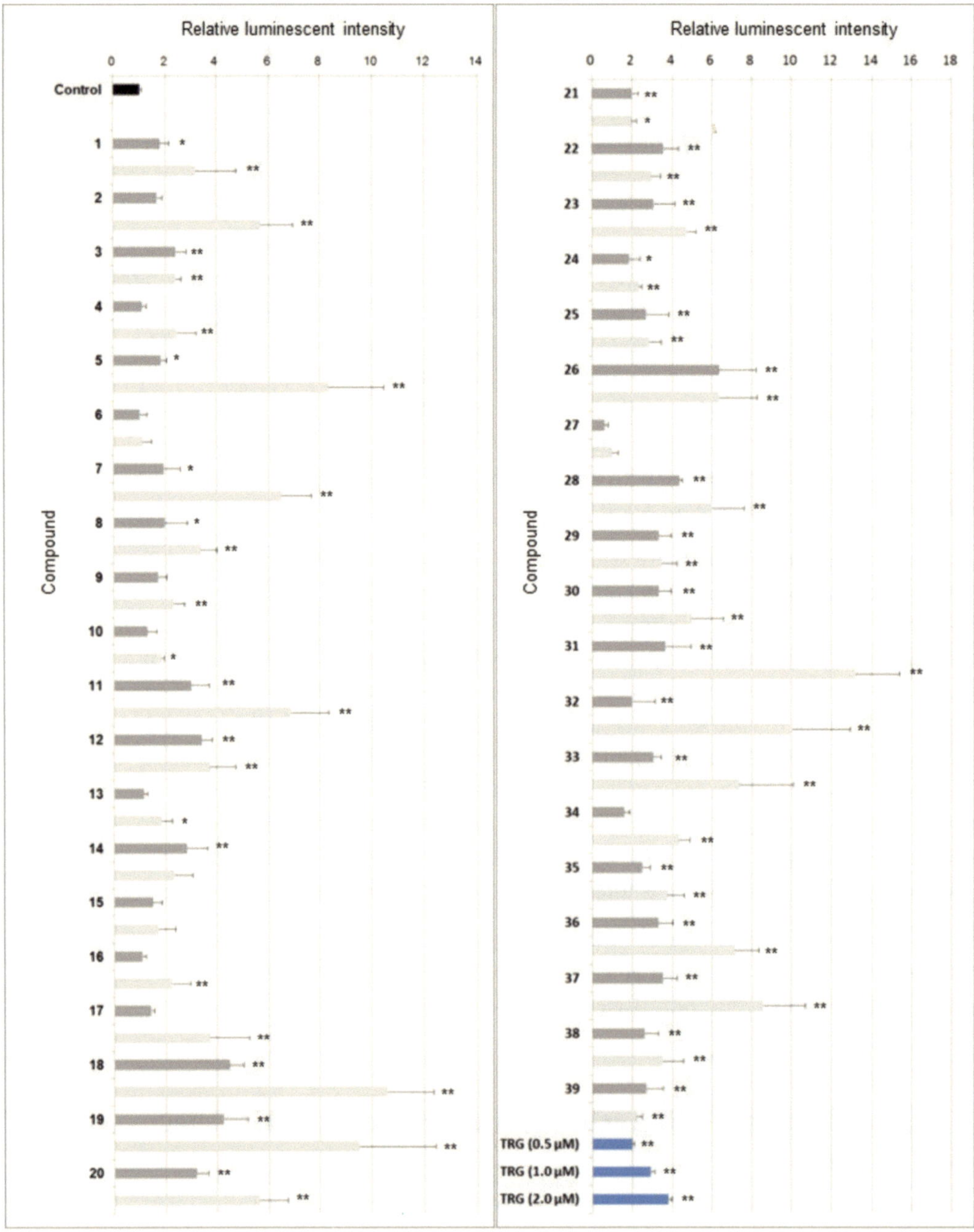

Figure 6. PPAR-γ ligand-binding activity of compounds **1–39** at 2 (■) and 10 ( ) μg/mL with a GAL-4-PPAR-γ chimera assay [1]. Troglitazone (TRG) at 0.5, 1.0, and 2.0 μM was used as a positive control, and dimethyl sulfoxide at 1 mL/L was used as a solvent control. Values are means ± SD, $n = 4$ experiments. Statistical significance is indicated by * ($p < 0.05$) or ** ($p < 0.01$) as determined by Dunnett's multiple comparison test.

that the two non-cyclic prenyl moieties were necessary for the potent activity of these compounds (**Figure 7**). Taking together all the above data, the PPAR-γ ligand-binding activity of the phenolic compounds was affected by slight differences in the substitution groups on the aromatic rings.

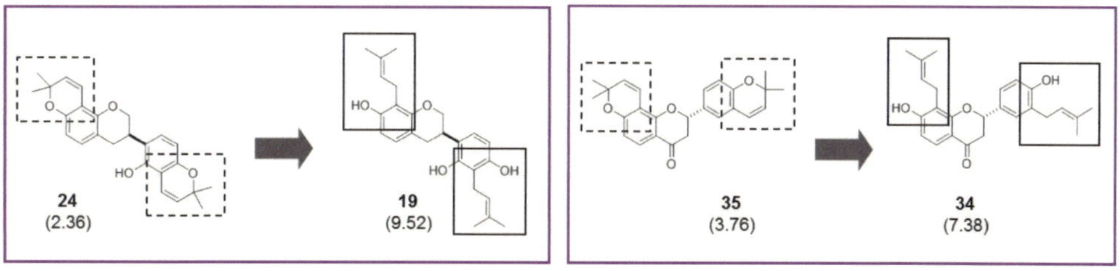

Figure 7. PPAR-γ ligand-binding activity of **19**, **24**, **34**, and **35** isolated from *G. glabra* roots [1]. Values in parentheses are the relative luminescence intensities at 10 μg/mL.

5. Isolation and structural determination of phenolic compounds from *G. uralensis*

The roots of *G. uralensis* (1.2 kg) were extracted with EtOAc (5.5 L) at room temperature for 7 days. The extract was then filtered and concentrated (74.0 g). The EtOAc extract of *G. uralensis* roots exhibited potent PPAR-γ ligand-binding activity and its relative luminescence intensity was 2.8 at a sample concentration of 30 μg/mL. This was almost equivalent to that of 1.0 μM TRG. The EtOAc extract was chromatographed on a silica gel column eluted with $CHCl_3$–MeOH gradients (19:1; 9:1; 4:1) and finally with MeOH to provide four fractions. PPAR-γ ligand-binding activity was concentrated in the $CHCl_3$-MeOH (19:1) eluate (relative luminescence intensity of 2.8 at 30 μg/mL). The $CHCl_3$-MeOH (19:1) eluate (55.4 g) was subjected to multiple chromatographic steps on a silica gel column eluted with $CHCl_3$-MeOH, an ODS silica gel column eluted with MeOH-H_2O and MeCN-H_2O, and to reversed phase HPLC using MeOH-H_2O and MeCN-H_2O mobile phases to obtain compounds **40–52** (22.2, 28.3, 58.7, 225, 80.7, 12.1, 43.5, 17.5, 11.8, 74.5, 51.0, 22.1, and 40.1 mg, respectively). Compounds **41–52** were identified by comparison of their physical and spectral data with those of reported compounds as dehydroglyasperin C (**41**) [28], glyasperin D (**42**) [29], glycycoumarin (**43**) [30], glycyrin (**44**) [31], glyasperin B (**45**) [29], glycyrol (**46**) [32], isoglycyrol (**47**) [32], glicoricone (**48**) [33], licoricone (**49**) [34], licocoumarone (**50**) [30], gancaonin I (**51**) [35], and liquiritigenin (**52**) [36] (**Figure 8**). This was the first isolation of glyasperin B (**45**) from *G. uralensis*. The structure of the new compound, **41**, was determined by 1D and 2D NMR spectroscopic analysis and

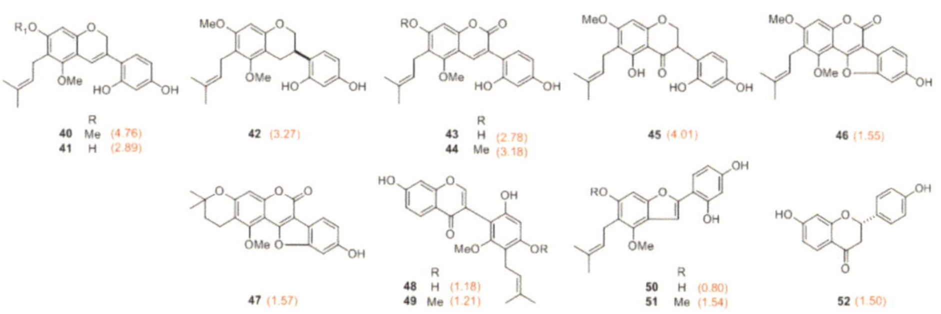

Figure 8. Structures of **40–52** isolated from *G. uralensis* roots [2]. Values in parentheses are the relative luminescence intensities at 5 μg/mL.

HRESIMS as 3-(2,4-dihydroxyphenyl)-5,7-dimethoxy-6-(3-methyl-2-butenyl)-2H-chromene and was named dehydroglyasperin D.

6. PPAR-γ ligand-binding activity of compounds 40–52 isolated from *G. uralensis*

Of the isolated compounds, the new compound **40** and known compounds **41–45** exhibited significant PPAR-γ ligand-binding activity (**Figure 6**). The activity of **40** at 5.0 μg/mL (=13.6 μM) was stronger than that of 2.0 μM TRG (relative luminescence intensity of 3.7). The coumestan derivative **46**, which was less active than **40**, was structurally similar to the active compound **43**, and the only detected difference between **43** and **46** was the formation of a five-membered ether ring between C-4 and C-2′ in **46**. This suggested that the presence of a hydroxy group at C-2′ in the isoflavan, isoflavene, or arylcoumarin skeleton is necessary for PPAR-γ ligand-binding activity. Furthermore, the isoflavones, **48** and **49**, which have a hydroxy group at C-2′ and no isoprenyl group at C-6, did not exhibit activity, suggesting that the isoprenyl group at C-6 was also involved in PPAR-γ ligand-binding activity. In conclusion, the isoprenyl group at C-6 and the C-2′ hydroxy group in the aromatic C ring of the isoflavan, isoflavene, or arylcoumarin skeleton were structural requirements for PPAR-γ ligand-binding activity (**Figure 9**).

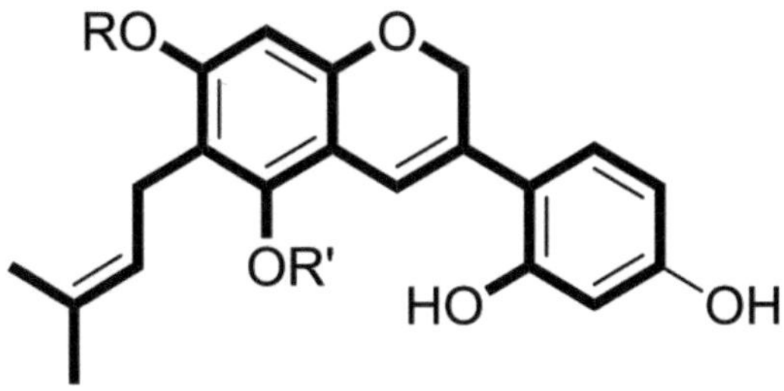

Figure 9. Structural requirements for the isoflavan skeleton for PPAR-γ ligand binding [2].

7. Ameliorative effects on diabetic KK-A^y mice

The ameliorative effects of glycyrin (**44**) in KK-A^y mice, an animal model of genetic type 2 diabetes, were studied using pioglitazone as a positive control. There was no difference in the food intake or body weight of mice between the treated groups and the control group. Test compound intake, calculated from the food intake and body weight of the mice, was approximately 100 mg/(kg day) in the glycyrin and glycyrol (**46**) groups and 23 mg/(kg day) in the pioglitazone group. Blood glucose levels significantly decreased after 4 days of feeding in both the glycyrin- and pioglitazone-treated groups compared to that in the control group, whereas the blood glucose levels of the glycyrol-treated group were comparable to those of the control group (**Table 1**).

	Control	Glycyrin (0.10%)	Glycyrol (0.10%)	Pioglitazone (0.02%)
Body weight (g)				
Day 0	52.6 ± 0.53	54.1 ± 1.78	52.6 ± 1.07	55.1 ± 0.69
Day 4	48.9 ± 0.48	50.4 ± 1.58	49.1 ± 1.02	53.6 ± 1.07
Day 7	50.4 ± 0.56	51.9 ± 1.62	50.3 ± 0.91	55.8 ± 1.50
Day 10	46.9 ± 0.42	48.1 ± 1.57	46.8 ± 0.08	52.5 ± 11.41
Average food intake (g/mouse/day)[b]	5.43	5.34	5.47	6.34
Average test compound intake (mg/kg/day)[c]	0	102	108	23
Blood glucose level (mg/dL)				
Day 0	476 ± 22	474 ± 27	427 ± 24	486 ± 26
Day 4	420 ± 14	278 ± 14**	421 ± 19	191 ± 6**

[a]Body weights and blood glucose levels are expressed as means ± SE of five mice.

[b]Calculated as (total food intake) (number of mice day).

[c]Calculated as (average food intake/average body weight of mice).

Statistical significance is indicated as ** ($P < 0.01$) as determined by Dunnett's multiple comparison test.

Table 1. Effect of feeding glycyrin (**44**) on KK-A^y mice in experiments for the preventing diabetes [2][a].

Pioglitazone, a potent PPAR-γ agonist that activates PPAR-γ, resulted in the improvement of insulin resistance and type 2 diabetes mellitus. Glycyrin exhibited significant PPAR-γ ligand-binding activity and appeared to reduce the blood glucose levels of KK-A^y mice by the same biological mechanism as pioglitazone. This finding was supported by the observation that glycyrol, structurally related to glycyrin but lacking PPAR-γ ligand-binding activity, failed to improve the hyperglycemia of KK-A^y mice.

8. Conclusion

Fractionation of the EtOH extract of *G. glabra* roots and the EtOAc extract of *G. uralensis* roots, guided by a GAL-4-PPAR-γ chimera assay method, resulted in the isolation of 52 phenolics, including 11 new compounds. The structures of the new compounds were determined by spectroscopic analysis. Of the isolated compounds, more than 10 phenolics exhibited significant PPAR-γ ligand-binding activity and the prenylflavone derivative, licoflavanone A (**31**), exhibited the most potent ligand-binding activity. The activity of these compounds at a sample concentration of 10 μg/mL was approximately three times greater than that of 0.5 μM TRG. Six phenolics were isolated from the EtOAc extract of *G. uralensis* roots as PPAR-γ ligands and one, glycyrin (**44**), reduced the blood glucose levels of genetically diabetic KK-A^y mice through its PPAR-γ ligand-binding activity. We have therefore discovered a possible new application of *G. glabra* and *G. uralensis* roots and their constituents for the amelioration of type 2 diabetes, a representative insulin resistance syndrome that is becoming a serious worldwide public health problem.

Author details

Minpei Kuroda* and Yoshihiro Mimaki

*Address all correspondence to: kurodam@toyaku.ac.jp

Department of Medicinal Pharmacognosy, School of Pharmacy, Tokyo University of Pharmacy and Life Sciences, Tokyo, Japan

References

[1] Kuroda M, Mimaki Y, Honda S, Tanaka H, Yokota S, Mae T. Phenolics from *Glycyrrhiza glabra* roots and their PPAR-γ ligand-binding activity. Bioorganic & Medicinal Chemistry 2010; 18: 962–970.

[2] Kuroda M, Mimaki Y, Sashida Y, Mae T, Kishida H, Nishiyama T, Tsukagawa M, Konishi E, Takahashi K, Kawada T, Nakagawa K, Kitahara M. Phenolics with PPAR-γ ligand-binding activity obtained from licorice (*Glycyrrhiza uralensis* Roots) and ameliorative effects of glycyrin on genetically diabetic KK-Ay mice. Bioorganic & Medicinal Chemistry Letters 2003; 13: 4267–4272.

[3] Takahashi N, Kawada T, Goto T, Yamamoto T, Taimatsu A, Matsui N, Kimura K, Saito M, Hosokawa M, Miyashita K, Fushiki T. Dual action of isoprenols on activation of both PPARγ and PPARα in 3 T3-L1 adipocytes and HepG2 hepatocytes. FEBS Letter 2002; 514: 315–322.

[4] The samples were dissolved in DMSO, to which the medium was added to obtain the final concentration of 0.1% (v/v) of DMSO. DMSO was also added to the control wells.

[5] Kajiyama K, Demizu S, Hiraga Y, Kinoshita K, Koyama K, Takahashi K, Tamura Y, Okada K, Kinoshita T. Two prenylated retrochalcones from *Glycyrrhiza inflate.* Pytochemistry 1992; 31: 3229–3232.

[6] Saitoh T, Shibata S. New type chalcone from licorice root. Tetrahedron Letters 1975; 16: 4461–4462.

[7] Delle Monache G, De Rosa M C, Scurria R, Vitali A, Cuteri A, Monacelli B, Pasqua G, Botta B. Comparison between metabolite productions in cell culture and in whole plant of *Maclura pomifera*. Phytochemistry 1995; 39: 575–580.

[8] Kinoshita T, Kajiyama K, Hiraga Y, Takahashi K, Tamura Y, Mizutani K. The isolation of new pyrano-2-arylbenzofuran derivatives from the root of *Glycyrrhiza glabra*. Chemical and Pharmaceutical Bulletin 1996; 44: 1218–1221.

[9] Ferrari F, Botta B, Alves de L R. Flavonoids and isoflavonoids from *Zollernia paraensis*. Phytochemistry 1983; 22: 1663–1664.

[10] Fukai T, Sheng C B, Horikoshi T, Nomura T. Isoprenylated flavonoids from underground parts of *Glycyrrhiza glabra*. Phytochemistry 1996; 43: 1119–1124.

[11] Gottlieb O.R., Braga de O.A., Goncalves T.M.M., De Oliveira G.G., Pereira S.A. Isoflavonoids from *Cyclolobium species*. Phytochemistry 1975; 14: 2495–2499.

[12] Song C, Zheng Z, Liu D, Hu Z. Antimicrobial isoflavans from *Astragalus membranaceus* (Fisch.) Bunge. Acta Botanica Sinica 1997; 39: 486–488.

[13] Saitoh T, Kinoshita T, Shibata S. New isoflavan and flavanone and licorice root. Chemical and Pharmaceutical Bulletin 1976; 24: 752–755.

[14] Mitscher L A, Park Y H, Omoto S, Clark G W, Clark D. Antimicrobial agents from higher plants, *Glycyrrhiza glabra* L. (var. *Spanish*). I. Some antimicrobial isoflavans, isoflavenes, flavanones and isoflavones. Heterocycles 1978; 9: 1533–1538.

[15] Kinoshita T, Kajiyama K, Hiraga Y, Takahashi K, Tamura Y, Mizutani K. Isoflavan derivatives from *Glycyrrhiza glabra* (Licorice). Heterocycles 1996; 43:581–588.

[16] Mitscher L A, Park Y H, Clark D, Beal J L. Antimicrobial agents from higher plants. Antimicrobial isoflavanoids and related substances from *Glycyrrhiza glabra* L. var. typica. Journal of Natural Products 1980; 43: 259–269.

[17] Kinoshita T, Tamura Y, Mizutani K. The isolation and structure elucidation of minor isoflavonoids from licorice of *Glycyrrhiza glabra* Origin. Chemical and Pharmaceutical Bulletin 2005; 53: 847–849.

[18] Kitagawa I, Chen W Z, Hori K, Harada E, Yasuda N, Yoshikawa M, Ren J. Chemical studies of Chinese licorice-roots. I. Elucidation of five new flavonoid constituents from the roots of *Glycyrrhiza glabra* L. collected in Xinjiang. Chemical and Pharmaceutical Bulletin 1994; 42: 1056-1062.

[19] Asada Y, Li W, Yoshikawa T. Isoprenylated flavonoids from hairy root cultures of *Glycyrrhiza glabra*. Phytochemistry 1998; 47: 389–392.

[20] Fukui H, Goto K, Tabata M. Two antimicrobial flavanones from the leaves of *Glycyrrhiza glabra*. Chemical and Pharmaceutical Bulletin 1988; 36: 4174–4176.

[21] Mizuno M, Tamura K, Tanaka T, Iinuma M. Six flavanones from the roots of *Euchresta formosana*. Phytochemistry 1989; 28: 2811–2812.

[22] Pereira M O da S, Fantine E C, De Sousa J R. Prenylated flavonoids from seeds of *Calopogonium mucunoides*. Phytochemistry 1982; 21; 488–489.

[23] Fukai T, Wang Q H, Takayama M, Nomura T. Structure of five new prenylated flavonoids L, M, N, O, and P from aerial parts of *Glycyrrhiza uralensis*. Heterocycles 1990; 31: 373–382.

[24] Kinoshita T, Saitoh T, Shibata S. The occurrence of an isoflavene and the corresponding isoflavone in licorice root. Chemical and Pharmaceutical Bulletin 1976; 24: 991–994.

[25] Nomura T, Fukai T. "Phenolic constituents of licorice (*Glycyrrhiza* Species)" in "Progress in the chemistry of organic natural products" Herz W, Kirby G W, Moore R E, Steglich W, Tamm C, Eds: Springer Wien: New York, 1998, Vol. 73, p. 27.

[26] Gaffield W. Circular dichroism, optical rotatory dispersion and absolute configuration of flavanones, 3-hydroxyflavanones and their glycosides: Determination of aglycone chirality in flavanone. Tetrahedron 1970; 26: 4093–4108.

[27] Kiuchi F, Chen X, Tsuda Y. Four new phenolic constituents from licorice (root of *Glycyrrhiza* sp.). Heterocycles 1990; 31: 629–636.

[28] Shibano M, Henmi A, Matsumoto Y, Kusano G, Miyase T, Hatakeyama Y. Studies on the index compounds for HPLC analysis of *Glycyrrhiza uralensis*. Heterocycles 1997; 45: 2053–2060.

[29] Zeng L, Fukai T, Nomura T, Zhang R Y, Lou Z C. Four new prenylated flavonoids, glyasperins A, B, C, and D from the roots of *Glycyrrhiza aspera*. Heterocycles 1992; 34: 575–587.

[30] Demizu S, Kajiyama K, Takahashi K, Hiraga Y, Yamamoto S, Tamura Y, Okada K, Kinoshita T. Antioxidant and antimicrobial constituents of licorice: Isolation and structure elucidation of a new benzofuran derivative. Chemical and Pharmaceutical Bulletin 1988; 36: 3474–3479.

[31] Kinoshita T, Saitoh T, Shibata S. A new 3-arylcoumarin from licorice root. Chemical and Pharmaceutical Bulletin 1978; 26: 135–140.

[32] Shiozawa T, Urata S, Kinoshita T, Saitoh T. Revised structures of glycyrol and isoglycyrol, constituents of the root of *Glycyrrhiza uralensis*. Chemical and Pharmaceutical Bulletin 1989; 37: 2239–2240.

[33] Hatano T, Fukuda T, Miyase T, Noro T, Okuda T. Phenolic constituents of licorice. III. Structures of glicoricone and licofuranone, and inhibitory effects of licorice constituents of monoamine oxidase. Chemical and Pharmaceutical Bulletin 1991; 39: 1238–1243.

[34] Saitoh T, Kinoshita T, Shibata S. Flavonols of licorice root. Chemical and Pharmaceutical Bulletin 1976; 24: 1242–1245.

[35] Fukai T, Wang Q H, Kitagawa T, Kusano K, Nomura T, Iitake Y. Structures of six isoprenoid-substituted flavonoids, gancaonins F, G, H, I, glycyrol, and isoglycyrol from Xibei licorice (*Glycyrrhiza* Sp.). Heterocycles 1989; 29: 1761–1772.

[36] Nakanishi T, Inada A, Kambayashi K, Yoneda K. Flavonoid glycosides of the roots of *Glycyrrhiza uralensis*. Phytochemistry 1985; 24: 339–341.

Chapter 6

Applicability of Licorice Extracts for Treatment of Oral Diseases, Evaluated by Simplified *In Vitro* Assay Systems with Oral Cells

Hiroshi Sakagami, Takao Kato, Kunihiko Fukuchi,
Taisei Kanamoto, Shigemi Terakubo,
Hideki Nakashima, Hirokazu Ohno and
Masaji Yamamoto

Additional information is available at the end of the chapter

http://dx.doi.org/10.5772/67435

Abstract

Licorice extracts contain various useful substances for oral health. Alkaline extract showed potent anti-HIV activity, whereas flavonoid-rich water extracts showed potent anti-HSV activity, closely correlated with polarizability, ionization potential, a number of ring systems, atomic number and mass. Licorice flavonoids showed higher tumor-specificity against human oral squamous cell carcinoma as compared with human normal oral mesenchymal cells. Glycyrrhiza, at noncytotoxic concentrations, potently inhibited the IL-1β-induced inflammation in cultured human gingival and periodontal ligament fibroblasts. Glycyrrhizin, a major component of Glycyrrhiza, showed the highest UV-protected activity. The results suggest the possible applicability of licorice extracts for several oral diseases and cosmetic products.

Keywords: herb extract, licorice, flavonoids, antiviral activity, tumor-specificity, anti-UV activity, anti-inflammatory activity, oral environment

1. Introduction

The oral cavity (mouth) includes the lips, cheeks, palate (roof of the mouth), floor of the mouth, and the part of the tongue in the mouth (oral tongue). The oral cavity is important for food digestion and speech, the taste buds for sensing different tastes, and the mouth for breathing, drinking, facial expressions, and social interactions.

It is now accepted that the improvement of oral environment leads to the enrichment of quality of life. The number of healthy teeth in aged people well correlates with longevity. In Japan, many of Kampo medicines and component herb extracts have been applied to various oral diseases. However, the selection of Kampo medicines in each case is mostly depended on the experiences of attending physicians, due to the absence of a quantitative evaluation method of their efficacy. This urged us to establish the quick *in vitro* quantification method of antiviral, antitumor, anti-inflammatory, and anti-UV activity, using appropriate cultured cells [1]. These methods were applied to various Kampo medicines and component extracts of plants including licorice to clarify their relative potency.

It was the best to use oral cells for the study of oral diseases. Therefore, we used oral squamous cell carcinoma cell lines and normal oral cells for the study of antitumor activity, and human gingival and periodontal ligament fibroblasts for the study of anti-inflammatory activity. However, we rather used nonoral cells for the study of antiviral and anti-UV activity due to their higher sensitivity (T-cell leukemia and Vero cells for HIV and HSV infection) and also considering the target specificity (skin cells for UV-irradiation).

2. Biological activity of licorice extracts and purified components

2.1. Preparation of flavonoid and chalcone derivatives

For the preparation of licorice flavonoids, the air-dried roots of *Glycyrrhiza inflate* were extracted with MeOH under reflux. The MeOH extracts were dried *in vacuo* and passed through a Diaion HP-20 column, eluting sequentially with H_2O, 50% EtOH and EtOH. The 50% EtOH eluate was chromatographed on a silica gel column ($CHCl_3$:MeOH:H_2O = 10:5:1) to give two fractions. The latter fraction was chromatographed on an octa decyl silyl (ODS) column (MeOH:H_2O, 45:55) to give three fractions. From the first fraction, liquiritin apioside, liquiritigenin 7-apiosylglucoside, liquiritin, and neoliquiritin were obtained with high-performance liquid chromatography (HPLC) (YMC-Pack Pro C18; MeOH:H_2O, 40:60 and CH_3CN:H_2O, 22:78). From the second fraction, isoliquiritin apioside, licurazid, isoliquiritin, and neoisoliquiritin were obtained with HPLC (YMC-Pack Pro C18, MeOH:H_2O, 50:50, and CH_3CN:H_2O, 30:70). From the third fraction, liquiritigenin and isoliquiritigenin were obtained with recycling HPLC (JAI-gel GS-310, MeOH) [2]. The structures of these compounds are shown in **Figure 1**.

For the preparation of water and alkaline extracts, the licorice roots (*Glycyrrhiza glabra* harvested in Afghanistan) were extracted for 20 h with water (not adjusted or adjusted to pH 9 or pH 12) at room temperature. These extracts were filtered through a membrane filter (pore size: 5 μm), neutralized with NaOH or H_2SO_4 and then dried to obtain the water extract (A), alkaline (pH 9.0) extract (B) and alkaline (pH 12.0) extract (C) at the yield of 18.0, 20.3, and 21.7%, respectively (**Figure 2A**). Two alkaline solutions (pH 9.0 and pH 12.0) extracted these ingredients at higher yield than water extraction. Glycyrrhizic acid was the most abundant compound in these extracts, followed by liquiritin apioside and licurazid (**Figure 2b**) [3].

http://dx.doi.org/10.5772/67435

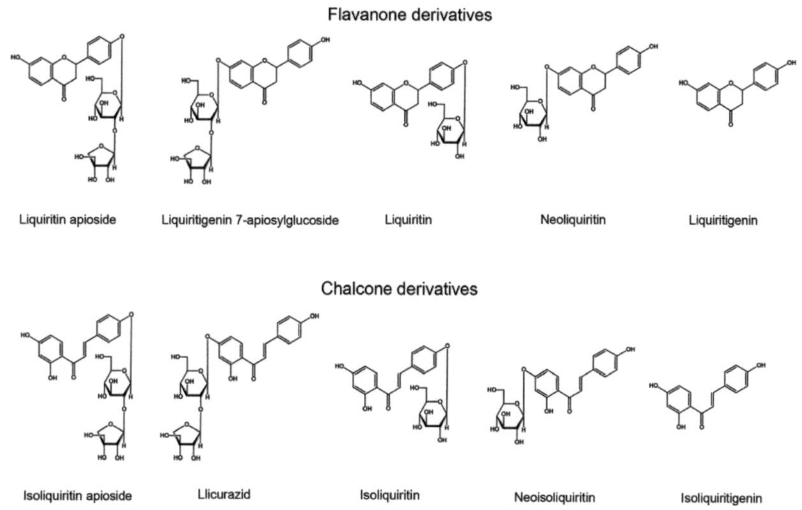

Figure 1. Structures of licorice root flavonoids.

A

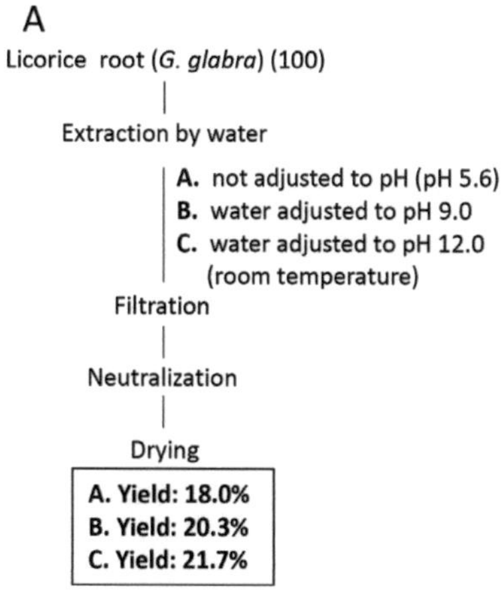

B

	Content (%)		
	Water extraction (A)	Alkaline extraction pH 9.0 (B)	pH 12.0 (C)
Glycyrrhizic acid	8.84	10.91	9.88
Liquiritin apioside	1.52	2.55	2.82
Liquiritigenin 7-apiosylglucoside	0.65	1.36	0.76
Liquiritin	0.38	0.74	0.42
Neoliquiritin	0.1	0.24	0.18
Liquiritigenin	0.16	0.13	0.09
Isoiquiritin apioside	0.93	0.9	0.34
Licurazid	1.81	1.1	2.47
Isoliquiritin	0.08	0.09	0.06
Neoisoliquiritin	0.06	0.05	0.11
Isoliquiritigenin	0.04	0.03	0.03

Figure 2. (A) Fractional preparation of water and alkaline extracts from licorice root (*G. glabra*) and distribution of major ingredients. (B) Major ingredients in each extract. Cited from Ref. [3].

2.2. Antiviral activity

2.2.1. *Anti-HIV activity*

Human T-cell leukemia virus I (HTLV-I)-bearing CD4-positive human T-cell line MT-4 was cultured in suspension in an RPMI-1640 medium supplemented with 10% FBS and infected with human immunodeficiency virus (HIV)-1_{IIIB} at a multiplicity of infection of 0.01. HIV- and mock-infected MT-4 cells were incubated for 5 days with different concentrations of extracts and the relative viable cell number was determined by MTT assay. The concentrations that reduced the viable cell number by 50% (CC_{50}) and that increased the number of viable HIV-infected cells to 50% of control (EC_{50}) were determined from the dose-response curve. The anti-HIV activity was evaluated by the selectivity index (SI) (SI = CC_{50}/EC_{50}). Infection of MT-4 cells with HIV-1 reduced the cell viability to almost zero. Alkaline extract of licorice root (*G. Glabra*) showed the protective effect on HIV infection (SI > 9.2), although its anti-HIV activity was much lower than that of anti-HIV agents [azidothymidine (AZT), 2′,3′-dideoxycytidine (ddC)] (SI = 3029–11,715) and an alkaline extract of the leaves of *Sasa senanensis* Rehder (SE) (SI = 42.7) (left column, **Table 1**). On the other hand, water extract of licorice root, flavonoid-rich fraction, glycyrrhizin acid, glycyrrhetinic acid, flavonoids (iquiritin apioside, liquiritin 7-apiosylglucose, liquiritin, neoliquiritin, liquiritigenin, isoliquiritin apioside, lucurzid, isoliquiritin, neoisoliquiritin, isoliquiritigenin), and polymethoxyflavonoids (tricin, 3,3′,4′,5,6,7,8-heptamethoxyflavone, nobiletin, tangeretin, sudachitin) were all inactive (SI < 1), due to their higher cytotoxicity [4].

	Anti-HIV activity (SI)	**Anti-HSV activity**			**Antitumor activity (TS)**	
		SI		**Maximum cell recovery (%)**	**Epithel. Tumor/ Mesen. normal (Method I)**	**Gingiva. Tumor/ Gingiva. normal (Method II)**
		Method I	**Method II**			
Licorice root extracts						
Water extract (μg/ml)	>1.3	><1	>4.6	60	><1	><1
Purified fraction of water extract (μg/ml)	<1	3.4	6.8	50	>3.5	4.2
Flavonoid-rich fraction of water extract (μg/ml)	<1	4.6	9.2	69	5.5	5.2
Water extract (different lot) (pH 5.6) (μg/ml)	><1	<1	2.0	57	><1	><1
Alkaline (pH 9.0) extract (μg/ml)	>3.0	<1	3.2	62	><1	><1
Alkaline (pH12.0) extract (μg/ml)	>9.2	<1	<1	49	><1	><1
Glycyrrhizin acid (μg/ml)	>1.2	<1	<1	ND	><1	><1
Glycyrrhetinic acid (μg/ml)	<1	<1	<1	ND	1.1	1.1
Licorice flavonoids						
Liquiritin apioside (μg/ml)	><1	>5	>500	79	><1.0	
Liquiritin 7-apiosylglucose (μg/ml)	><1	><1	>21	58	1.0	
Liquiritin (μg/ml)	<1	<1	2.8	55	>1.7	
Neoliquiritin (μg/ml)	<1	<1	2.9	59	><0.9	
Liquiritigenin (μg/ml)	<1	2.4	>6	77	2.0	

http://dx.doi.org/10.5772/67435

	Anti-HIV activity (SI)	Anti-HSV activity			Antitumor activity (TS)	
		SI		Maximum cell recovery (%)	Epithel. Tumor/ Mesen. normal (Method I)	Gingiva. Tumor/ Gingiva. normal (Method II)
		Method I	Method II			
Isoliquiritin apioside (μg/ml)	><1	23.1	>455	82	><1.1	
Lucurzid (μg/ml)	><1	><1	>667	65	9.0	
Isoliquiritin (μg/ml)	<1	21.4	128.6	97	2.2	
Neoisoliquiritin (μg/ml)	<1	8.0	10.9	87	><0.9	
Isoliquiritigenin (μg/ml)	<1	<1	2.0	54	4.4	
Licochalcone A (μg/ml)					2.0	
Polymethoxyflavonoids						
Tricin (μM)	<1	5.8	7.0	67	><1.0	><1.0
3,3',4',5,6,7,8-Heptamethoxyflavone (μM)	<1	<1	1.1	50	2.0	2.8
Nobiletin (μM)	<1	<1	<1	42	2.0	1.8
Tangeretin (μM)	<1	<1	<1	45	3.0	2.4
Sudachitin (μM)	<1	<1	<1	42	2.9	1.7
Positive control						
AZT (μM)	11,715					
ddC (μM)	3029					
Epigallocatechin gallate (μM)		<1	4.7	62		
Chlorogenic acid (μM)		<1	<1	49		
Coumaric acid (μM)		<1	<1	69		
Curcumin (μM)		1.9	ND	75		
Resveratrol (μM)		<1	2.8	55		
Doxorubicin (μM)					69.9	54.8
5-FU (μM)					>8.9	>28.8
Methotexate (μM)					>170	>45
SE (%)	42.7	8.7	10.2	100	1.6	1.5

Table 1. Anti-HIV, anti-HSV, and antitumor activity of licorice extracts. Cited from Ref. [4].

Ten Kampo medicine and 25 constituent herb extracts showed little or no anti-HIV activity (SI = 1–4) (**Table 2**) [15], possibly due to the fact that most of them were prepared by hot water extraction.

Name	Glycyrrhizin content (mg/g)	LPS contamination (ng/g)	Anti-UV activity (SI)		Anti-HIV activity SI
			HSC-2	HaCaT	
Constituent herb extracts					
Alisma rhizome	<0.1	<2	><1.0	11	><1.0
Asiasarum root	<0.1	2	><1.0	>13	<1.0
Astragalus root	<0.1	17	><1.0	>13	><1.0
Atractylodes lancea rhizome	<0.1	16	<0.8	<0.1	>1.9
Bupleurum root	<0.1	17	<0.7	<0.1	><1.0
Cimicifuga rhizome	<0.1	15	>1.4	9.7	<1.0
Cinnamon bark	<0.1	13	<0.6	7.1	<1.0
Cnidium rhizome	<0.1	18	><1.0	>9.2	>1.5
Coptis rhizome	<0.1	16	1.5	13	<1.0
Gardenia fruit	<0.1	15	>8	>23	>2.7
Ginger	<0.1	14	<0.8	<0.3	><1.0
Ginseng	<0.1	18	><1.0	>7.1	><1.0
Glycyrrhiza	175.4	19	4.3	4.4	<1.0
Japanese Angelica root	<0.1	18	><1.0	>3.9	>1.1
Japanese Gentian	<0.1	16	>1.1	>20	><1.0
Jujube	<0.1	16	><1.0	>3	><1.0
Peony root	<0.1	16	><1.0	>18	<1.0
Phellodendron bark	<0.1	14	<0.1	10	<1.0
Pinellia tuber	<0.1	<2	><1.0	>3.7	><1.0
Platycodon root	<0.1	18	<0.8	<0.15	><1.0
Polyporus sclerotium	<0.1	19	>1.0	>26	>4.4
Poria sclerotium	<0.1	<2	><1.0	4.8	><1.0
Rehmannia root	<0.1	10	><1.0	>7.1	><1.0
Saposhnikovia root	<0.1	13	>1.3	>20	><1.0
Scutellaria root	<0.1	<2	<0.9	38	<1.0
Chinese medicines					
Byakkokaninjinto	7.2	17	><1.0	3.5	<1.0
Hangesyashinto	16.2	9	>4.9	>28	<1.0

http://dx.doi.org/10.5772/67435

Name	Glycyrrhizin content (mg/g)	LPS contamination (ng/g)	Anti-UV activity (SI)		Anti-HIV activity SI
			HSC-2	HaCaT	
Hotyuekkito	0.2	11	><1.0	>5.1	><1.0
Juzentaihoto	7	18	><1.0	>9.6	<1.0
Kikyoto	50.3	18	1.05	4.4	<1.0
Ninjinyoeito	3.5	19	><1.0	23	><1.0
Rikkosan	24.1	>200	>1.2	>6.8	<1.0
Saireito	7	17	>3.4	>19	<1.0
Shosaikoto	9.2	19	>4.3	34	<1.0
Unseiin	<0.1	>200	>4.9	>23	<1.0
Glycyrrhizin		<1	20.6	36.4	>2.0
Vitamin C			44	200	
AZT					17,850

Table 2. Anti-UV and anti-HIV activity of Kampo medicine and constitutional plant extract. Cited from Refs. [15, 16].

2.2.2. *Anti-HSV activity*

We have recently established the simple *in vitro* assay method of antiherpes simplex virus (HSV) activity. Vero cells, isolated from the kidney of African green monkey (*Cercopithecus aethiops*), [5] were infected with HSV-1 (multiplicity of infection = 0.01). First, HSV-1 and test samples were mixed and stood for 20 min, and the mixture was then added to the adherent Vero cells. After incubation for 4 days, the relative viable cell number was quantified by MTT reagent to yield CC_{50}, EC_{50}, and selectivity index (SI) (SI = CC_{50}/EC_{50}). By infection with HSV-1, the cell viability dropped to 34.1 ± 8.9% (18.3–51.1%) (n = 33). Addition of licorice root extracts recovered the cell density to 51–64% of control level. The incomplete recovery of cell viability urged us to adopt the following two methods for measuring EC_{50}. In method 1, EC_{50} was defined as the concentration at which the viability was restored to the midpoint between that of HSV-infected cells and that of mock-infected cells. In method II, EC_{50} was defined as the concentration at which the viability was restored to 50% that of mock-infected cells (see example in **Figure 3**) [4].

It was unexpected that water extract of licorice root [SI = >< 1 (method I); 4.6 (method II)] showed higher anti-HSV activity than alkaline extract (pH 12) (SI < 1 and < 1). Among water extracts, flavonoid-rich fraction showed the highest anti-HSV activity (SI = 4.6; 9.2). Among licorice flavonoids, liquiritin apioside (SI >5; >500), isoliquiritin apioside (SI >23.1; >455), lucurzid (SI >< 1; >667) and isoliquiritin (SI = 21.4; 128.6) showed the highest anti-HSV activity (center column in **Table 1**).

Among five polymethoxyflavonoids, the SI value for tricin (SI = 5.8; 7.0) (**Figure 1**) was comparable with that of SE, while the other four polymethoxyflavonoids (3,3′,4′,5,6,7,8-heptamethoxyflavone, nobiletin, tangeretin, sudachitin) had little or no anti-HSV activity

(SI < 1; < 1–1.1) (**Table 1**). Among lower molecular polyphenols, epigallocatechin gallate, a major compound in green tea, had some anti-HSV activity (SI < 1; 4.7), followed by resveratrol (SI < 1; 2.8).

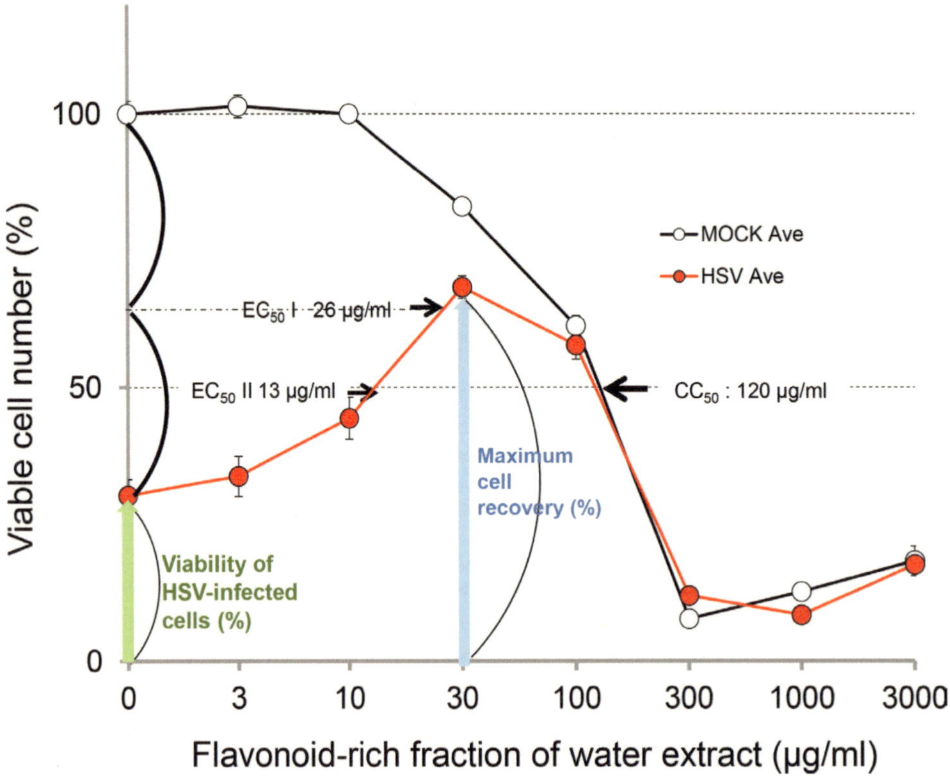

Figure 3. Anti-HSV activity of flavonoid-rich fraction of water extract of liquorice root. Each value represents the mean ± SD of triplicate assays. The 50% effective concentration (EC_{50}), determined by method I or II (see **Table 2**), and 50% cytotoxic concentration (CC_{50}) is indicated by arrows. Cited from Ref. [4]. Cited from Ref. [3].

The quantitative structure-activity relationship (QSAR) analysis [4] demonstrated that anti-HSV activity of licorice flavonoids and lower molecular weight polyphenols correlated well with six chemical descriptors that represent polarizability (MATS5p, GATS5p) [6, 7], ionization potential (GATS5i) [7], a number of ring systems (NRS) [8], and atomic number (J_Dz(Z)) and mass (J_Dz(m) [9] ($r^2 = 0.684, 0.627, 0.624, 0.621, 0.619$ and 0.618, respectively, $p < 0.0001$) (**Figure 4**). This result suggests that the physicochemical properties, rather than the category of compound, are important for determining anti-HSV activity.

2.3. Antitumor activity

The tumor-selectivity index (TS) was calculated by dividing the mean CC_{50} against normal cells by the mean CC_{50} against tumor cells. We used the following two methods. Method I:

human gingival fibroblast (HGF) + human periodontal fibroblast (HPLF) + human pulp cells (HPC) (normal mesenchymal cells) versus Ca9-22 + HSC-2 + HSC-3 + HSC-4 (human oral squamous cell carcinoma) (epithelial cells). Method II: HGF (gingival normal mesenchymal cells) versus Ca9-22 (gingival tumor epithelial cells) [10] (**Table 1**). We have confirmed that the TS value reflects the antitumor activity, based on the finding that antitumor drugs have extremely higher TS values [11].

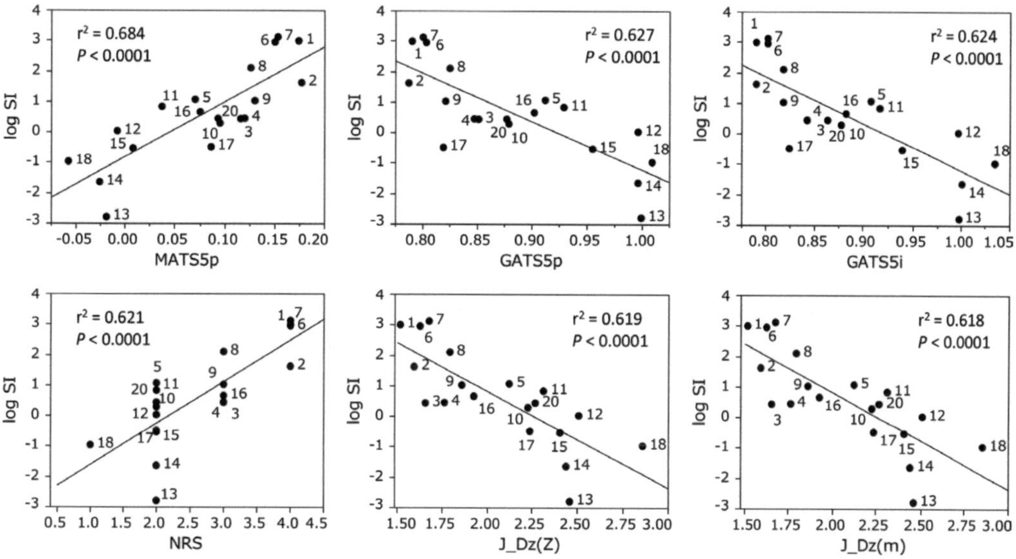

Figure 4. QSAR analysis of anti-HSV activity (defined as SI value determined by method II) of licorice flavonoids, polymethoxyflavonoids, and low molecular weight flavonoids. The log SI value was calculated from -logCC_{50} value and -logEC_{50} value. 1, liquiritin apioside; 2, liquiritin 7-apiosylglucose; 3, liquiritin; 4, neoliquiritin; 5, liquiritingenin; 6, isoliquiritin apioside; 7, lucurzid; 8, isoliquiritin; 9, neoisoliquiritin; 10, isoliquiritigenin; 11, tricin; 12, 3,3′,4′,5,6,7,8-heptamethoxyflavone; 13, nobiletin; 14, tangeretin; 15, sudachitin; 16, epigallocatechin gallate; 17, chlorogenic acid; 18, coumaric acid; 20, resveratrol. The data of curcumin, 19, was not included since the SI value could not be obtained (center column, **Table 1**). Cited from Ref. [4].

Among licorice root extracts, flavonoid-rich fraction of water extract showed the highest TS [TS = 5.5 (method I); 5.2 (method II)], although this value was much lower than that of popular antitumor drugs (doxorubicin, 5-fluorouracil, methotrexate, melphalan: TS = 8.9–170). Among licorice flavonoids, neoisoliquiritin apioside and isoliquiritigenin exhibited the highest antitumor activity (TS = 4.4–9.0), which was well correlated with their solvation energy ($r^2 = 0.659$) (QSAR analysis) [2]. Five polymethoxyflavonoids (tricin, 3,3′,4′,5,6,7,8-heptamethoxyflavone, nobiletin, tangeretin, and sudachitin) were weakly tumor selective (TS = 1.0–3.0) (right column, **Table 1**) [4].

2.4. Anti-inflammatory activity

We found that interleukin (IL)-1β stimulated the production of prostaglandin (PG)E_2, interleukin (IL)-6, IL-8, and monocyte chemoattractant protein-1 (MCP-1) by human gingival fibroblast (HGF) to much higher extent than that achieved by LPS prepared from *Escherichia coli* and *Porphyromonas gingivalis* [12]. Glycyrrhiza extract significantly inhibited the IL-1β-stimulated PGE_2 production by HGF cells (EC_{50} = 95 μg/ml, CC_{50} > 4000 μg/ml; SI = CC_{50}/EC_{50} > 22) (**Figure 5A**). Similarly, glycyrrhiza extract significantly inhibited the IL-1β-stimulated PGE_2 production by human periodontal ligament fibroblasts (HPLF) cells (EC_{50} = 32 μg/ml, CC_{50} = 1878 μg/ml; SI = CC_{50}/EC_{50} = 59) (**Figure 5B**) [13]. The endospecy test with LAL reagent revealed that LPS contamination in glycyrrhiza and glycyrrhizin was very low (19 ng/g and <1 ng/g, respectively) (**Table 2**) [14].

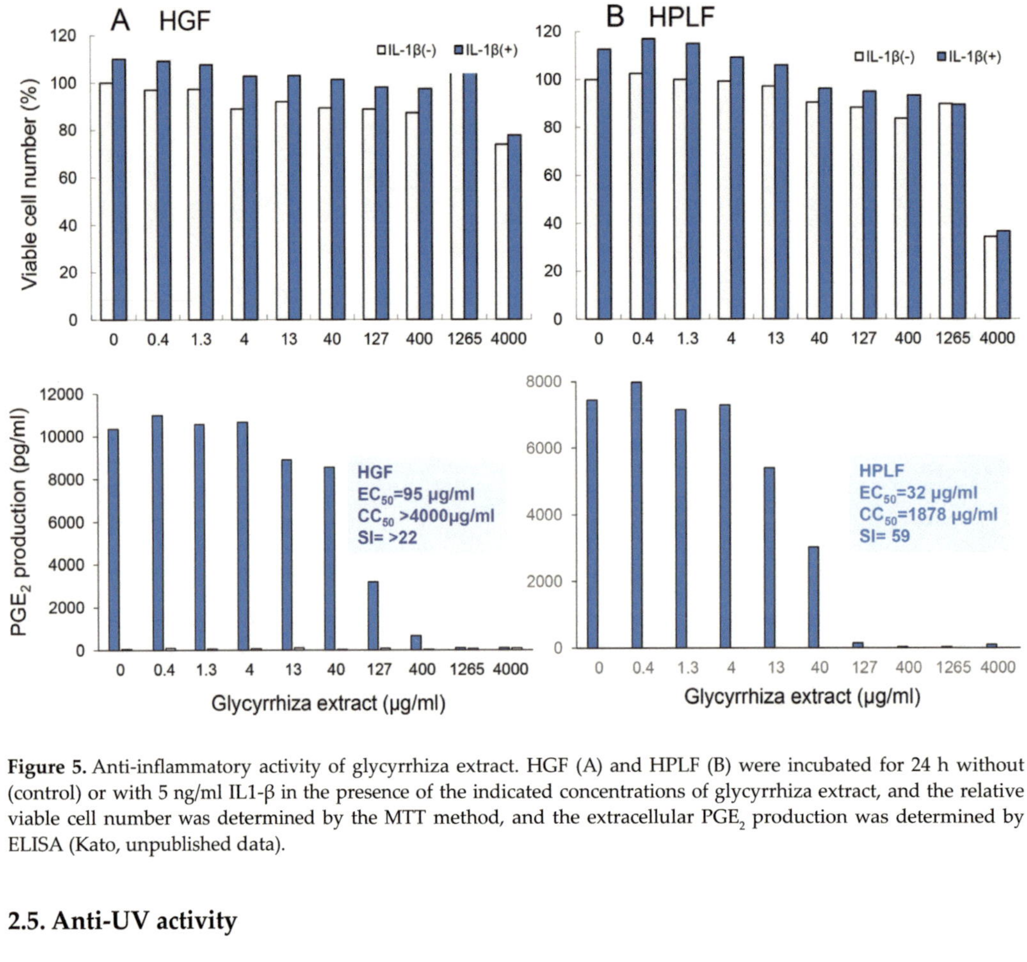

Figure 5. Anti-inflammatory activity of glycyrrhiza extract. HGF (A) and HPLF (B) were incubated for 24 h without (control) or with 5 ng/ml IL1-β in the presence of the indicated concentrations of glycyrrhiza extract, and the relative viable cell number was determined by the MTT method, and the extracellular PGE_2 production was determined by ELISA (Kato, unpublished data).

2.5. Anti-UV activity

We measured the ability of test samples to protect the UV-induced injury (referred to as anti-UV activity), using UV-sensitive cell line HSC-2 cell. We found that glycyrrhizin, a major component of Glycyrrhiza, exhibited very high anti-UV activity (SI = 20.6) (**Figure 6A, Table 2**). In order to determine whether there is any correlation of anti-UV activity and glycyrrhizin content, we investigated the concentration of glycyrrhizin in the plant extracts and Kampo medicines by HPLC [JASCO PU-980 pump, a JASCO UV-970 UV/VIS detector, Inertsil ODS-3 column, 254 nm; mobile phase: 2.5% acetic acid (40: 60)]. Twenty-five plant extracts, except for Glycyrrhiza (175.4 mg/g), did not contain detectable amounts of glycyrrhizin, whereas 10

http://dx.doi.org/10.5772/67435

Kampo medicines (Byakkokaninjinto, Hangesyashinto, Hotyuekkito, Juzentaihoto, Kikyoto, Ninjinyoeito, Rikkosan, Saireito, Shosaikoto, Unseiin) contained up to 50.3 mg/g of glycyrrhizin, possibly due to the inclusion of Glycyrrhiza (**Table 2**). However, there was no clear-cut relationship between the anti-UV activity and glycyrrhizin content of Kampo medicines and constituent plant extracts [15] (**Table 2**).

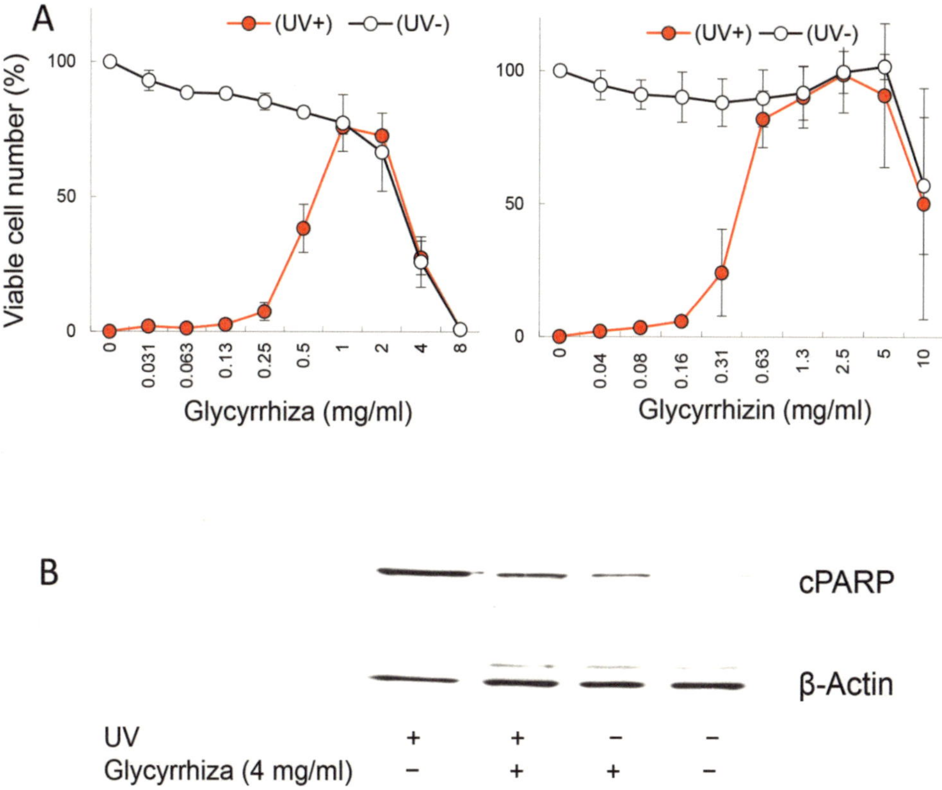

Figure 6. (A) Anti-UV activity of glycyrrhiza (left) and glycyrrhizin (right), (B) protective effect of glycyrrhiza on the UV-induced apoptosis in HSC-2 cells (western blot analysis). Cited from Ref. [15].

Western blot analysis demonstrated that UV irradiation induced the production of cleaved PARP, indicating the activation of caspase-3/-7 in HSC-2 cells, and that glycyrrhiza inhibited the UV-induced caspase activation (**Figure 6B**).

Since it is preferable to use skin-derived cells for the determination of anti-UV activity, we investigated the anti-UV activity of Kampo medicines using human immortal skin keratinocyte cell line HaCaT. We found that the HaCaT cell system gave nearly 1 order higher SI value than the HSC-2 system, maintaining good correlation of anti-UV activity measured between these two cell lines ($r^2 = 0.33$) (**Figure 7A**). There was some correlation between the anti-UV activity (defined as SI value) and absorbance at 253.7 nm in both systems ($r^2 = 0.14$ and 0.24, respectively) (**Figure 7B**), suggesting that some part of anti-UV activity comes from the direct absorption of UV.

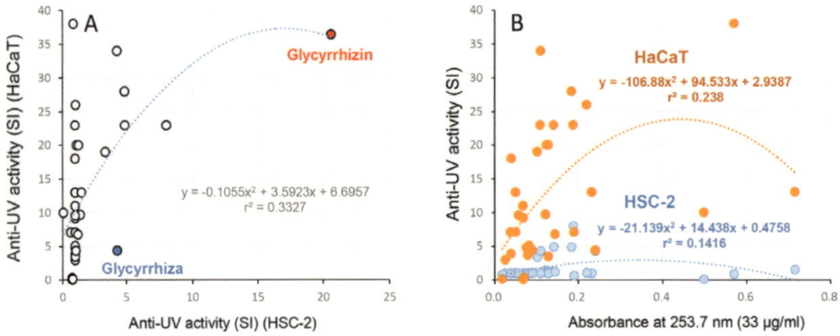

Figure 7. (A) Correlation between anti-UV activities measured in HSC-2 cells and that in HaCaT cells. (B) The correlation of anti-UV activity and absorbance (optical density) measured at 253.7 nm (Kato et al., unpublished data).

Among 10 Kampo medicines, Shosaikoto (SI = 34) showed the highest anti-UV activity, followed by Hangesyashinto (SI > 28), Unseiin (SI > 23), Ninjinyoeito (SI = 23), and Saireito (SI > 19), whereas other four Kampo medicines were much less active (SI < 9.6) (**Table 2**). Among 25 plant extracts, Scutellaria root exhibited the highest anti-UV activity (SI = 38), followed by Polyporus sclerotium (SI > 26), Gardenia fruit (SI > 23), Japanese Gentian (SI > 20), and Saposhnikovia root (SI > 20). Glycyrrhizin also exhibited potent anti-UV activity (SI = 36) (**Table 2**) [16].

3. Conclusions

Alkaline extract of licorice roots showed greater anti-HIV activity than the water extract, while the water extract, especially the flavonoid-rich fraction, showed greater anti-HSV activity than the alkaline extract (**Table 1**), suggesting that water and alkaline extracts might show different site of actions against these two viruses.

It was unexpected that five polymethoxyflavonoids including tricin showed very low level of anti-HSV activity (**Table 1**), since tricin has been reported to show a broad antiviral spectrum [17–20]. It remains to be investigated whether the combination of these compounds with acyclovir [5] or ganciclovir [21] may increase viability of infected cells.

The present study also demonstrated that neoisoliquiritin apioside showed the highest antitumor activity. Isoliquiritin has been reported to inhibit granuloma angiogenesis and tube formation in vascular endothelial cells [22]. Further studies are required to elucidate the mechanism by which this compound induces such high tumor specificity.

We have recently reported that titanium dioxide nanoparticles (TiO_2 NPs) were incorporated into vacuoles of HGF cells and aggravated the gingival inflammation (characterized by the enhanced prostaglandin E_2 production and COX-1 and COX-2 protein expression, and the reduction of intracellular concentrations of amino acid, urea cycle, polyamine, *S*-adenosylmethione and glutathione synthetic pathways) [23]. This finding recommends carful use of dental materials containing TiO_2 NPs for patients with gingivitis or periodontitis. It remains to be investigated whether glycyrrhiza extracts or their fractions can neutralize the aggravation effects of TiO_2 NPs.

More than 80 reports have investigated the anti-inflammatory effect of Kampo medicines (reviewed in Refs. [24] and [25]). However, basic research and clinical studies for the treatment of oral diseases are much less [26–30], and little is known about the relative potency of Kampo medicines. Potent antiviral, anti-inflammatory, antitumor, and anti-UV activities of licorice extracts, demonstrated here, suggest their possible applicability for treating several oral diseases and manufacturing cosmetic products.

QSAR analysis is a useful technique to predict the most active three-dimensional structure. The next step is to synthesize the compound with predicted structure and then investigate the biological activity. This prediction-synthesis-confirmation cycle should be repeated until obtaining the expected biological activity (**Figure 8**). The applicability of such compounds on oral diseases should be tested.

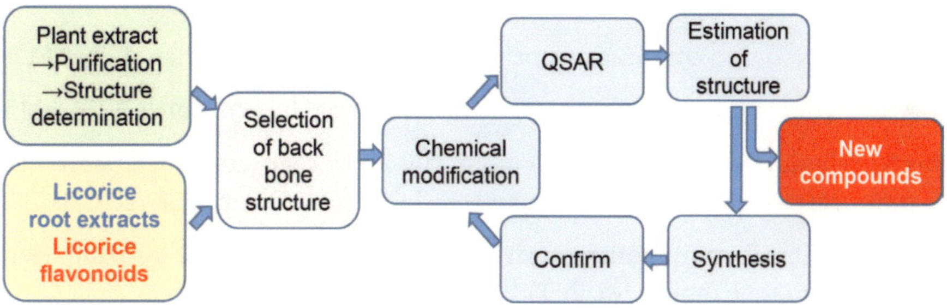

Figure 8. Scheme of manufacturing new anti-HSV agents from licorice extracts.

Author details

Hiroshi Sakagami[1,*], Takao Kato[2], Kunihiko Fukuchi[3], Taisei Kanamoto[4], Shigemi Terakubo[4], Hideki Nakashima[4], Hirokazu Ohno[5] and Masaji Yamamoto[5]

*Address all correspondence to: sakagami@dent.meikai.ac.jp

1 Division of Pharmacology, Meikai University School of Dentistry, Japan

2 Department of Oral and Maxillofacial Surgery, Kanazawa Medical University, Japan

3 Graduate School, Showa University, Tokyo, Japan

4 St. Marianna University School of Medicine, Kanagawa, Japan

5 Research Center, Maruzen Pharmaceuticals Co., Ltd., Japan

References

[1] Sakagami H: Biological activities and possible dental application of three major groups of polyphenols. J Pharmacol Sci. 2014;**126**:92–106.

[2] Ohno H, Araho D, Uesawa Y, Kagaya H, Ishihara M, Sakagami H, Yamamoto M: Evaluation of cytotoxicity and tumor-specificity of licorice flavonoids based on chemical structures. Anticancer Res. 2013;**33**:3061–3068.

[3] Ohno H, Miyoshi S, Araho D, Kanamoato T, Terakubo S, Nakashima H, Tsuda T, Sunaga K, Amano S, Ohkoshi E, Sakagami H, Satoh K, Yamamoto M: Efficient utilization of licorice root by alkaline extraction. In Vivo. 2014;**28**:785–794.

[4] Fukuchi K, Okudaira N, Adachi K, Odai-Ide R, Watanabe S, Ohno H, Yamamoto M, Kanamoto T, Terakubo S, Nakashima H, Uesawa Y, Kagaya H, Sakagami H: Antiviral and antitumor activity of licorice root extracts. In Vivo. 2016;**30**:777–786.

[5] Sakagami H, Fukuchi K, Kanamoto T, Terakubo S, Nakashima H, Natori T, Suguro-Kitajima M, Oizumi H, Yasui T, Oizumi T: Synergism of alkaline extract of the leaves of *Sasa senanensis* Rehder and antiviral agents. In Vivo. 2016;**30**:421–426.

[6] Moran PAP: Notes on continuous stochastic phenomena. Biometrika. 1950;**37**:17–23.

[7] Geary RC: The contiguity ratio and statistical mapping. Incorp Statist. 1954;**5**:115–145.

[8] Feher M, Schmidt JM: Property distributions: differences between drugs, natural products, and molecules from combinatorial chemistry. J Chem Inf Comput Sci. 2003;**43**:218–227.

[9] Ivanciuc O: QSAR comparative study of Wiener descriptors for weighted molecular graphs. J Chem Inf Comput Sci. 2000;**40**:1412–1422.

[10] Horikoshi M, Kimura Y, Nagura H, Ono T, Ito H: A new human cell line derived from human carcinoma of the gingiva. I. Its establishment and morphological studies. (in Japanese). Japan J Oral Maxillofac Surg. 1974;**20**:100–106.

[11] Suzuki R, Matsuo S, Sakagami H, Okada Y, Shirataki Y: Search of new cytotoxic crude materials against human oral squamous cell carcinoma using NMR metabolomics Anticancer Res. 2014;**34**:4117–4120.

[12] Ono M, Kantoh K, Ueki J, Shimada A, Wakabayashi H, Matsuta T, Sakagami H, Kumada H, Hamada N, Kitajima M, Oizumi H, Oizumi T: Quest for anti-inflammatory substances using IL-1β-stimulated gingival fibroblasts. In Vivo. 2011;**25**:763–768.

[13] Kato T, Segami N, Sakagami H: Anti-inflammatory action of Kampo medicines and component herb extracts in relation to LPS contamination. (In Japanese). 2015 132th Kanto Regional Meeting, the Japanese Pharmacological Society, Chiba, July 2015.

[14] Kato T, Segami N, Sakagami H: Anti-inflammatory activity of hangeshashinto in IL-1β-stimulated gingival and periodontal ligament fibroblasts. In Vivo. 2016;**30**:257–264.

[15] Kato T, Horie N, Matsuta T, Umemura N, Shimoyama T, Kaneko T, Kanamoto T, Terakubo S, Nakashima H, Kusama K, Sakagami H: Anti-UV/HIV activity of Kampo medicines and constituent plant extracts. In Vivo. 2012;**26**:1007–1013.

[16] Kato T, Hino S, Horie N, Shimoyama T, Kaneko T, Kusama K, Sakagami H: Anti-UV activity of Kampo medicines and constituent plant extracts: re-evaluation with skin keratinocyte system. In Vivo. 2014;**28**:571–578.

[17] Wang HK, Xia Y, Yang ZY, Natschke SL, Lee KH: Recent advances in the discovery and development of flavonoids and their analogues as antitumor and anti-HIV agents. Review Adv Exp Med Biol. 1998;**439**:191–225.

[18] Matsuta T, Sakagami H, Satoh K, Kanamoto T, Terakubo S, Nakashima H, Kitajima M, Oizumi H, Oizumi T. Biological activity of luteolin glycosides and tricin from *Sasa senanensis* Rehder. In Vivo. 2011;**25**:757–762.

[19] Murayama T, Li Y, Takahashi T, Yamada R, Matsubara K, Tuchida Y, Li Z, Sadanari H. Anti-cytomegalovirus effects of tricin are dependent on CXCL11. Microbes Infect. 2012;**14**:1086–1092.

[20] Yazawa K, Kurokawa M, Obuchi M, Li Y, Yamada R, Sadanari H, Matsubara K, Watanabe K, Koketsu M, Tuchida Y, Murayama T. Anti-influenza virus activity of tricin, 4′,5,7-trihydroxy-3′,5′-dimethoxyflavone. Antivir Chem Chemother. 2011;**22**:1–11.

[21] Yamada R, Suda H, Sadanari H, Matsubara K, Tuchida Y, Murayama T: Synergistic effects by combination of ganciclovir and tricin on human cytomegalovirus replication in vitro. Antiviral Res. 2016;**125**:79–83.

[22] Kobayashi S, Miyamoto T, Kimura I, Kimura M: Inhibitory effect of isoliquiritin, a compound in licorice root, on angiogenesis in vivo and tube formation in vitro. Biol Pharm Bull. 1995;**18**: 1382–1386.

[23] Garcia-Contreras R, Sugimoto M, Umemura N, Kaneko M, Hatakeyama Y, Soga T, Tomita M, Scougall-Vilchis RJ, Contreras-Bulnes R, Nakajima H, Sakagami H: Alteration of metabolomic profiles by titanium dioxide nanoparticles in human gingivitis model. Biomaterials. 2015;**57**:33–40.

[24] Xia Q, Zhang H, Sun X, Zhao H, Wu L, Zhu D, Yang G, Shao Y, Zhang X, Mao X, Zhang L and She G: A comprehensive review of the structure elucidation and biological activity of triterpenoids from Ganoderma spp. Molecules. 2014;**30**:17478–17535.

[25] Shen Y, Li CG, Zhou SF, Pang EC, Story DF, Xue CC: Chemistry and bioactivity of Flos Magnoliae, a Chinese herb for rhinitis and sinusitis. Review. Curr Med Chem. 2008;**15**:1616–1627.

[26] Hijikata Y, Makiura N, Kano T, Higasa K, Shimizu M, Kawata K, Mine T: Kampo medicine, based on traditional medicine theory, in treating uncured glossodynia: efficacy in five clinical cases. Am J Chin Med. 2008;**36**:853–847.

[27] Liao J, Zhao L, Yoshioka M, Hinode D, Grenier D: Effects of Japanese traditional herbal medicines (Kampo) on growth and virulence properties of Porphyromonas gingivalis and viability of oral epithelial cells. Pharm Biol. 2013;**51**:1538–1544.

[28] Ara T, Honjo K, Fujinami Y, Hattori T, Imamura Y, Wang PL: Preventive effects of a Kampo medicine, orento on inflammatory responses in lipopolysaccharide treated human gingival fibroblasts. Biol Pharm Bull. 2010;**33**:611–616.

[29] Ohshima S, Hatori Y, Honma S, Terasawa K, Saitoh Y, Kobayashi D: Analysis of body constitution of 52 patients with Stevens-Johnson Syndrome (SJS) using Kampo medical questionnaires: prediction of SJS based on body constitution using decision tree. Yakugaku Zasshi. 2011;**131**:745–756.

[30] Sharma R, Tobin P, Clarke SJ. Sharma R, Tobin P, Clarke SJ: Management of chemotherapy-induced nausea, vomiting, oral mucositis, and diarrhoea. Lancet Oncol. 2005;**6**: 93–102.

Chapter 7

In Vitro Fertilization Activators for Future

Hiromitsu Tanaka, Morimasa Wada,
Nguyen Huu Tung, Shunsuke Fujii,
Takuhiro Uto and Yukihiro Shoyama

Additional information is available at the end of the chapter

http://dx.doi.org/10.5772/66317

Abstract

Artificial insemination is an indispensable technology for cattle breeding and is used for treating infertility in humans. Thus, new or improved methods are needed to increase the efficiency of artificial insemination. *In vitro* fertilization (IVF) has been developed in mice. Although many mouse lines produced using IVF have been preserved by freezing embryos and/or fertilized eggs, the more efficient IVF using freezing preservation or long-term refrigeration of sperm is expected to preserve mouse lines more easily. In this chapter, we introduce the active compounds in licorice to improve the rate of IVF. We previously reported that the rate of IVF in mice was improved by adding a water extract of licorice (*Glycyrrhiza uralensis*), but not glycyrrhizin, to the artificial insemination culture medium. Recently, we analyzed the active ethyl acetate fraction containing high levels of flavonoids. This fraction was further purified by bioassay-guided separation to isolate isoliquiritigenin and formononetin, which contributed to the improved rate of IVF. Isoliquiritigenin and formononetin may be useful therapeutic agents for infertility treatment.

Keywords: *in vitro* fertilization, activator, licorice, isoliquiritigenin, formononetin

1. Introduction

Glycyrrhiza species (Leguminosae), commonly known as licorice, are perennial plants that grow up to 1.5 m high and are distributed in drylands from Western Europe to Russia, and are particularly abundant in China and Mongolia. Licorice mainly consists of dried roots and stolons of *G. uralensis* Fisch and *G. glabra* Linne. Therefore, two species are listed in pharmacopoeia worldwide. Licorice is one of the most important crude drugs prescribed with other herb medicines in traditional Chinese medicine (TCM) for the treatment and prophylaxis of sore throats (as an antitussive), coughs and bronchial catarrh (as an expectorant), inflammation, allergic reactions, rheumatism and arthritis, liver disease, tuberculosis and adrenocorticoid insufficiency [1–5]. Nearly 500 components have been identified in licorice. Among them, glycyrrhizin is controlled at a concentration of more than 2.0% as a standardization marker component because the phamacological properties of licorice might be depend upon glycyrrhizin, and furthermore a flavonoid liquiritin has a quantitative limitation in Japanese pharmacopoeia [1]. Glycyrrhizin is a protein-kinase inhibitor with anti-ulcer and anti-viral activities [6]. In Japan and China, nowadays, glycyrrhizin is used for the treatment of hepatitis [4, 7–9]. It has been reported that glycyrrhizin has interferon-inducing activity and anti-HIV-1 activity [10–12]. Moreover, glycyrrhizin is well known as a natural sweetener and used in food additives and cosmetics [13]. On the other hand, flavonoids have also various pharmacological activities such as anti-hepatotoxic, anti-inflammatory, anti-ulcer, anti-allergenic and anti-viral as well as cardioprotective activities [2]. **Figure 1** indicates major components in licorice.

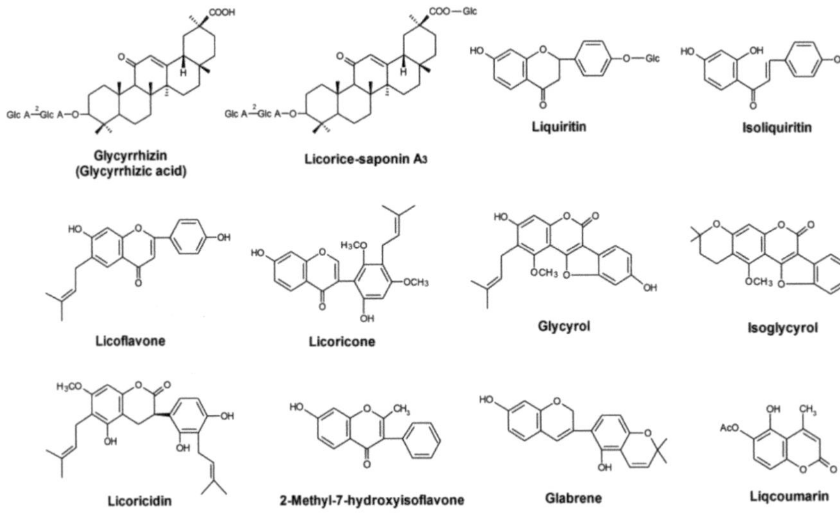

Figure 1. Major components in licorice.

In order to control the quality of licorice, we investigated and succeeded the preparation of monoclonal antibody (MAb) against glycyrrhizin and set up an enzyme-linked immunosorbent assay (ELISA) as quick, simple and reproducible assay system [14]. Furthermore, a new staining system, eastern blotting was developed [15] and immunoaffinity isolation of glycyrrhizin resulting in glycyrrhizin-knockout extract, which can be used to survey the real activity of glycyrrhizin in licorice [16, 17]. Regarding flavonoid, anti-liquiritin MAb [18] and eastern blotting [19] was developed. Since the above knowledge of components in licorice have been accumulated and also Tanaka et al. have been investigating about proteins [20–22] and mitochondria [23] related to fertilization using reproducing assay system, we have started to survey *in vitro* fertilization (IVF) active components in licorice.

2. *In vitro* fertilization of mouse sperm by licorice crude extract and fraction

Although previous studies have investigated whether licorice can increase pregnancy rates or not, the clear result has not been found yet [24]. However, since it is known that glycyrrhizin acts as the modulator of 11β-hydroxysteroid dehydrogenase (Type 1 and 2) which are the enzyme related to steroidal hormone [25], a speculation of relationship between licorice and testosterone and/or estrogen comes out. In fact Hajirahimkhan et al. searched three licorice species, *G. uralensis*, *G. glabra* and *G. inflata*, and found that isoliquiritigenin indicated strong estrogen-like activity, suggesting that this compound may be cyclized to liquiritigenin, which is an active flavonoid, under physiological conditions [26].

The sperm from wild-type C57BL/6 mice has high capacity for fertilization when cultured in standard medium (e.g., HTF) supplemented with bovine serum albumin for IVF or with polyvinyl alcohol (PVA) and methyl β-cyclodextrin (MBCD). On the other hand, IVF efficiency using the sperm of aged BALB/cA mice (>48 weeks of age) is low, albeit fluctuated between mice [27]. However, we found that the licorice crude extract improved the fertilizing ability of BALB/cA mouse sperm *in vitro* as indicated in **Figure 2** and that the fertilized eggs developed normally [28]. We performed five separate experiments using five different BALB/cA mice. The fertilization rate for HTF medium containing PVA plus MBCD and licorice extract (0.12 mg/ml) was between 15.6 and 84.0% (average: 43.0 ± 11.0%). On the other hand, the fertilization rate was between 0.0 and 43.5% (average: 15.0 ± 7.8%) when licorice extract-free medium was used. The optimal concentration of licorice extract in HTF medium was 0.3 mg/ml.

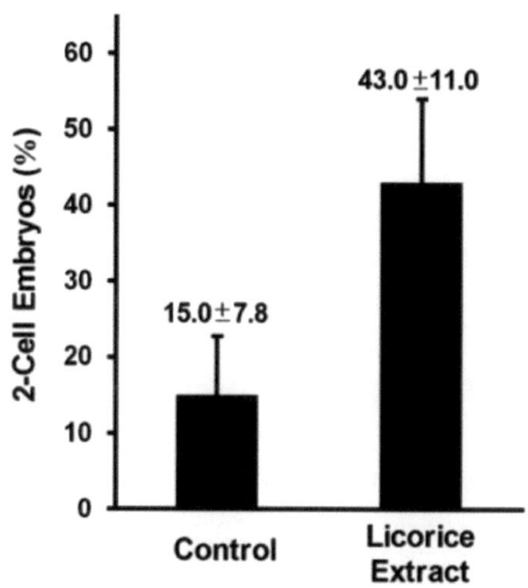

Figure 2. Influence of licorice extract on the IVF. Sperm from BALB/cA mice was preincubated in conditioned medium with or without licorice extract (0.12 mg/mL). Two-cell embryos were effectively obtained with preincubation medium containing licorice extract. The extract had a significant effect on IVF ($n = 5$, $P < 0.05$).

Park et al. reported that licorice extract increased cyclophosphamide teratogenicity and upregulated the mRNA expression of cytochrome P-450 2B in rats [29]. The results suggest that licorice root contains various bioactive components. However, they may not affect gene expression because transcription rates in spermatozoa are low [30]. Our findings indicate that components in licorice other than glycyrrhizin, or together other components and glycyrrhizin, can improve the IVF rates without damaging fertilized eggs.

In order to confirm the property of active component in licorice, the crude extract was fractionated with EtOAc and *n*-BuOH successively. **Figure 3** showed the fertilization level indicated by the percentage of two-cell embryos describing that the EtOAc fraction was more effective compared to that of *n*-BuOH fraction. From this result, active components might be not conjugated compounds like saponins including glycyrrhizin but free compound like flavonoids as indicated in **Figure 1** depending on their solubility.

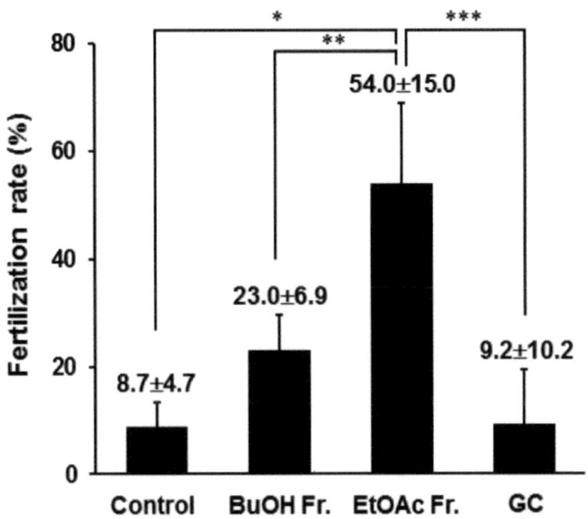

Figure 3. Active fraction of licorice extract and glycyrrhizin against IVF. *n*-BuOH (1.6 mg/mL) and EtOAc (1 mg/mL) fractions of licorice and glycyrrhizin (1.6 mg/mL) were added to the conditioned medium. Activity was observed in the EtOAc fraction containing flavonoids.

3. Survey of active components in licorice

The above active EtOAc fraction was bioassay-guided separated by silica gel column chromatography with a $CHCl_3$-MeOH solvent system as an eluent to give five fractions (1–5). Fraction 2 was further purified using a reversed-phase C18 column eluting with MeOH-H_2O to yield active compound **1**. Fraction 4 was also purified by the same way of fraction 2 to give active compound **2**.

Compound **1** was a yellow powder indicating an ion peak at *m/z* 257 $[M+H]^+$ in mass spectrometry having strong yellow fluorescence. From these evidences, compound **1** was supposed to be a non-conjugated flavonoid like a chalcone derivative, which has strong fluorescence in general. Finally, compound **1** was determined to be isoliquiritigenin (**Figure 4**) [31] by ^{13}C

nuclear magnetic resonance (NMR), 1-dimensional (1D; ^{1}H and ^{13}C) and 2D correlation spectroscopy (COSY), heteronuclear multiple quantum coherence (HMQC) and heteronuclear multiple-bond coherence (HMBC) spectroscopies.

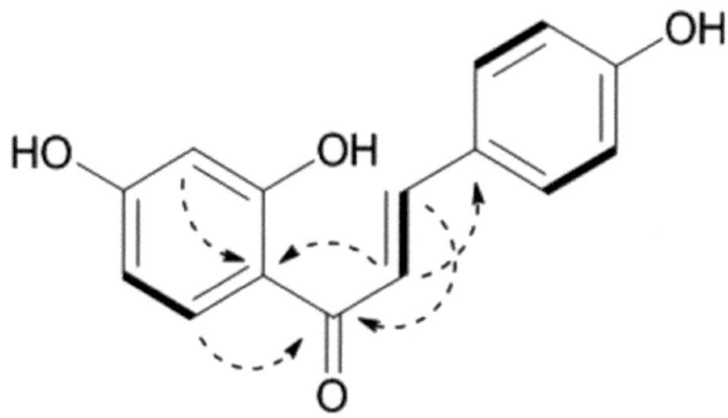

Figure 4. The structures of isoliquiritingenin with key COSY (bold lines) and HMBC correlations (dash arrows).

Compound **2** was a pale yellow powder indicating an ion peak at *m/z* 268 $[M+H]^{+}$ that the mass fragment pattern resembled to a flavonoid compound having a methoxyl group in a molecule. ^{13}C NMR showed a typical lower-shifted C-3 carbon (124.9 *m/z*) suggesting that compound **2** might be an isoflavone. The spectra of ^{1}H, ^{13}CNMR and 2D (COSY, HMQC and HMBC) confirmed that compound **2** was formononetin [32] (**Figure 5**).

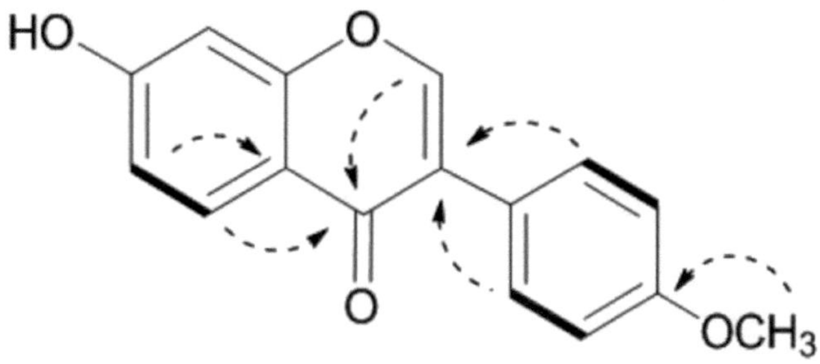

Figure 5. The structures of formononetin with key COSY (bold lines) and HMBC correlations (dash arrows).

4. Confirmation of IVF activity for two isolated components

The HTF medium containing PVA and MBCD with isoliquiritigenin or formononetin at a concentration range from 0 to 0.04 mg/ml was tested for IVF [33]. The optimal concentration of isoliquiritigenin was found at 0.02 mg/ml resulting in 47.2 ± 16.8% of IVF ratio. In the case of forononetin, the ratio was slightly higher (50.2 ± 9.5%) but not significantly, than that of isoliquiritigenin as indicated in **Figure 6**.

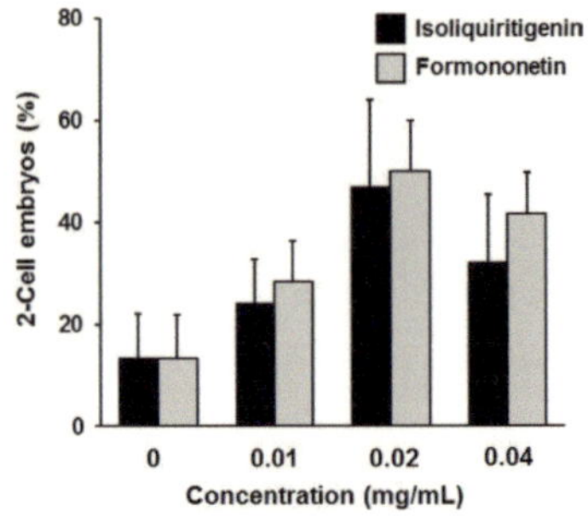

Figure 6. Optimal concentration of licorice extract for IVF. Black and gray bars indicated isoliquiritigenin and formononetin, respectively.

We examined the viability of embryos treated with isoliquiritigenin (**Figure 7A**) or formononetin (**Figure 7B**) to confirm that both embryos were morphologically normal similar to the previous observations using licorice crude extract [28].

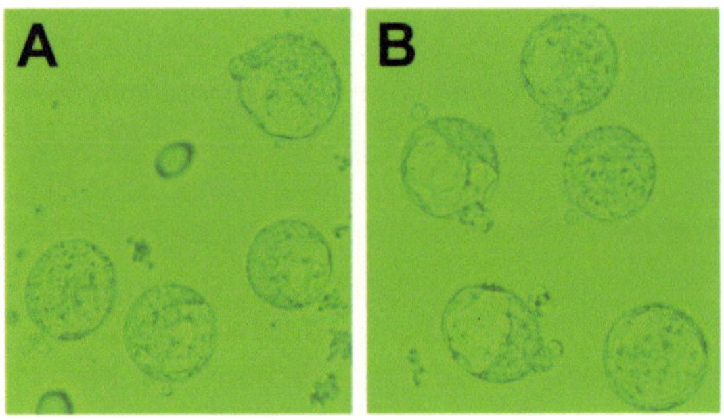

Figure 7. Morphology of blastocysts incubated with isoliquiritigenin or formononetin.

5. Licorice in future

It is considered that the decrease of population is now a serious problem in advanced countries depending on diversification of course of life (late marriage, unmarried, etc.). Carlsen et al. reported interesting evidence related to human semen [34]. It became evident that approximately 30% decrease of sperm number during 40 years from 1950 to 1990 occurred. From this data, it suggested that the number of sperm was half in 2005 compared to that in 1950. This evidence may be deeply related to the decrease of population. In order to increase the fertilization ratio, the activation of sperm is necessary against the decrease of sperm number and also the mechanism of increase of IVF by isoliquiritigenin or formononetin should be evident.

We investigated the incorporation and distribution of isoliquiritigenin or formononetin in mice sperm in order to obtain some information related to the mechanism. **Figure 8** showed the fluorescence staining in mice sperm using fluorescence microscope. Staining distributed in

http://dx.doi.org/10.5772/66317

almost all part of sperm. It seems to be that this phenomenon might be related to activation of sperm although the mechanism is still unknown and should be solved from now.

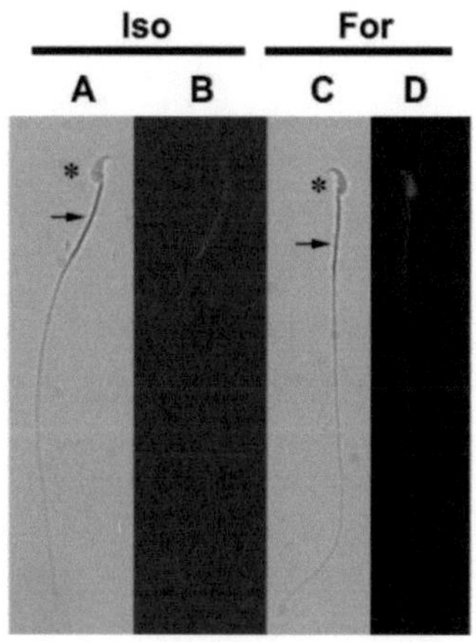

Figure 8. Fluorescence imaging of mice sperm in the preincubation medium with isoliquiritigenin (Iso) and formononetin (For). Signals were observed intensely in postacrosomal region (star) and mid piece (arrow).

Licorice used to be used for approximately 70% of TCM formula. From this current status, the pseudohyperaldosteronism often occurred by over uptake of licorice. It is well known that this phenomenon was occurred by taking of much glycyrrhizin. Glycyrrhizin is hydrolyzed to give glycyrrhetic acid (aglycone) by enteric bacteria, resulting the reabsorption of glycyrrhetic acid. This compound is changed to mono glycoside in liver. Glycyrrhetic acid monoglycoside inhibits 11β-hydroxysteroid dehydrogenase (HSD), which catalyzes the conversion of cortisol to cortisone resulting in the accumulation of cortisol which reacts to aldosterone receptor.

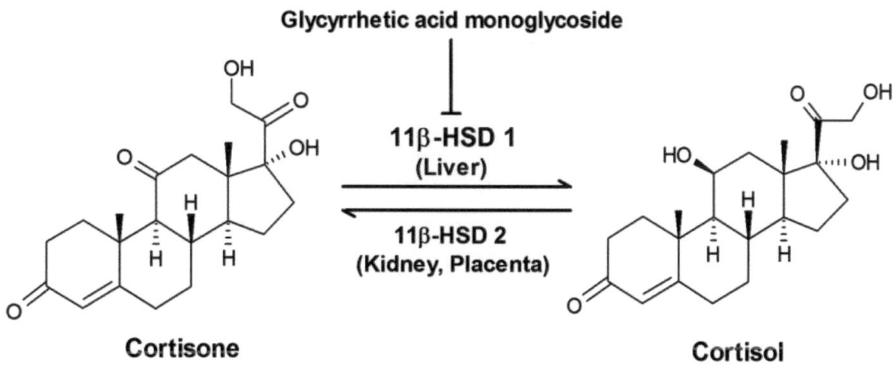

Figure 9. The inhibition of 11β-hydroxsteroid dehydrogenase (HSD) by glycyrrhetic acid monoglycoside inhibits in liver.

This phenomenon activates the reabsorption of sodium ion, and on the other hand potassium ion is eliminated inducing pseudohyperaldosteronism. Therefore, if we take too much licorice extracts for promotion of fertilization, such disease may be occurred. Previously, we purified glycyrrhizin from the crude extract of licorice using an immunoaffinity column conjugated with anti-glycyrrhizin monoclonal antibody, and prepared glycyrrhizin-knockout extract [17]. The glycyrrhizin-knockout extract contains all components except glycyrrhizin. Thus, glycyrrhizin-knockout extract can function for promoting fertilization **Figure 9**.

Author details

Hiromitsu Tanaka, Morimasa Wada, Nguyen Huu Tung, Shunsuke Fujii, Takuhiro Uto and Yukihiro Shoyama*

*Address all correspondence to: shoyama@niu.ac.jp

Faculty of Pharmaceutical Sciences, Nagasaki International University, Huis Ten Bosch, Sasebo, Nagasaki, Japan

References

[1] Taira Z, Yabe K, Hamaguchi Y, Hirayama K, Kishimoto M, Ishida S, Ueda Y. Effects of Sho-saiko-to extract and its components, Baicalin, baicalein, glycyrrhizin and glycyrrhetic acid, on pharmacokinetic behavior of salicylamide in carbon tetrachloride intoxicated rats. Food Chem Toxicol. 2004;42(5):803–807.

[2] Kim SC, Byun SH, Yang CH, Kim CY, Kim JW, Kim SG. Cytoprotective effects of *Glycyrrhizae* radix extract and its active component liquiritigenin against cadmium-induced toxicity (effects on bad translocation and cytochrome c-mediated PARP cleavage). Toxicology. 2004;197(3):239–251.

[3] Fuchikami J, Isohama Y, Sakaguchi M, Matsuda M, Kucota T, Akie YK, Fujino A, Miyata T. Effect of glycyrrhizin on late asthmatic responses induced by antigen inhalation in guinea pigs. J Pharmacol Sci. 2004;94(Suppl.1): 251.

[4] Jakkula M, Boucher TA, Beyendorff U, Conn SM, Johnson JE, Nolan CJ, Peine CJ, Albrecht JH. A randomized trial of Chinese herbal medicines for the treatment of symptomatic hepatitis C. Arch Intern Med. 2004;164(12):1341–1346.

[5] Yanagawa Y, Ogura M, Fujimoto E, Shono S, Okuda E. Effects and cost of glycyrrhizin in the treatment of upper respiratory tract infections in members of the Japanese maritime self-defense force: preliminary report of a prospective, randomized, double-blind, controlled, parallel-group, alternate-day treatment assignment clinical trial. Curr Ther Res Clin Exp. 2004;65(1):26–33.

[6] Hsiang CY, Lai IL, Chao DC, Ho TY. Differential regulation of activator protein 1 activity by glycyrrhizin. Life Sci. 2002;70(14):1643–1656.

[7] Xu J, Tanaka H, Shoyama Y. One-step immunochromatographic separation and ELISA quantification of glycyrrhizin from traditional Chinese medicines. J Chromatogr B Analyt Technol Biomed Life Sci. 2007;850(1–2):53–58.

[8] Lian Z, Niwa K, Gao J, Tagami K, Mori H, Tamaya T. Association of cellular apoptosis with anti-tumor effects of the Chinese herbal complex in endocrine-resistant cancer cell line. Cancer Detect Prev. 2003;27(2):147–154.

[9] Chung WT, Lee SH, Kim JD, Sung NS, Hwang B, Lee SY, Yu CY, Lee HY. Effect of the extracts from *Glycyrrhiza uralensis* Fisch on the growth characteristics of human cell lines: anti-tumor and immune activation activities. Cytotechnology. 2001;37(1):55–64.

[10] Davidson A, Siddell S. Potential for antiviral treatment of severe acute respiratory syndrome. Curr Opin Infect Dis. 2003;16(6):565–571.

[11] Cinatl J, Morgenstern B, Bauer G, Chandra P, Rabenau H, Doerr HW. Glycyrrhizin, an active component of liquorice roots, and replication of SARS-associated coronavirus. Lancet. 2003;361(9374):2045–2046.

[12] Bedoya LM, Palomino SS, Abad MJ, Bermejo P, Alcami J. Screening of selected plant extracts for *in vitro* inhibitory activity on human immunodeficiency virus. Phytother Res. 2002;16(6):550–554.

[13] Kim NC, Kinghorn AD. Highly sweet compounds of plant origin. Arch Pharm Res. 2002;25(6):725–746.

[14] Tanaka H, Shoyama Y. Formation of a monoclonal antibody against glycyrrhizin and development of an ELISA. Biol Pharm Bull. 1998;21(12):1391–1393.

[15] Shan S, Tanaka H, Shoyama Y. Enzyme-linked immunosorbent assay for glycyrrhizin using anti-glycyrrhizin monoclonal antibody and an eastern blotting technique for glucuronides of glycyrrhetic acid. Anal Chem. 2001;73(24):5784–5790.

[16] Uto T, Tuvshintogtokh I, Shoyama Y. Preparation of knockout extract for determination of really active compound using MAb. Curr Drug Discov Technol. 2011;8(1):16–23.

[17] Uto T, Morinaga O, Tanaka H, Shoyama Y. Analysis of the synergistic effect of glycyrrhizin and other constituents in licorice extract on lipopolysaccharide-induced nitric oxide production using knock-out extract. Biochem Biophys Res Commun. 2012;417(1): 473–478.

[18] Fujii S, Morinaga O, Uto T, Nomura S, Shoyama Y. Development of a monoclonal antibody-based immunochemical assay for liquiritin and its application to the quality control of licorice products. J Agric Food Chem. 2014;62(15):3377–3383.

[19] Fujii S, Morinaga O, Uto T, Nomura S, Shoyama Y. Development of double eastern blotting for major licorice components, glycyrrhizin and liquiritin for chemical quality control of licorice using anti-glycyrrhizin and anti-liquiritin monoclonal antibodies. J Agric Food Chem. 2016;64(5):1087–1093.

[20] Kitamura K, Nishimura H, Nishimune Y, Tanaka H. Identification of human HAPRIN potentially involved in the acrosome reaction. J Androl. 2005;26(4):511–518.

[21] Tanaka H, Iguchi N, Toyama Y, Kitamura K, Takahashi T, Kaseda K, Maekawa M, Nishimune Y. Mice deficient in the axonemal protein Tektin-t exhibit male infertility and immotile-cilium syndrome due to impaired inner arm dynein function. Mol Cell Biol. 2004;24(18):7958–7964.

[22] Tokuhiro K, Isotani A, Yokota S, Yano Y, Oshio S, Hirose M, Wada M, Fujita K, Ogawa Y, Okabe M, Nishimune Y, Tanaka H. OAZ-t/OAZ3 is essential for rigid connection of sperm tails to heads in mouse. PLoS Genet. 2009;5(11):e1000712.

[23] Nakada K, Sato A, Yoshida K, Morita T, Tanaka H, Inoue S, Yonekawa H, Hayashi J, Mitochondria-related male infertility related to fertilization, PNAS. 2006;103(41) 15148–15153.

[24] Shin S, Jang JY, Choi BI, Baek IJ, Yon JM, Hwang BY, Park D, Jeon JH, Nam SY, Yun YW, Kim YB. Licorice extract does not impair the male reproductive function of rats. Exp Anim. 2008;57(1):11–17.

[25] Yaw HP, Ton SH, Kadir KA. Glycyrrhizic acid as the modulator of 11β-hydroxysteroid dehydrogenase (type 1 and 2) in rats under different physiological conditions in relation to the metabolic syndrome. J Diabetes Metab. 2015;6:522.

[26] Hajirahimkhan A, Simmler C, Yuan Y, Anderson JR, Chen SN, Nikolić D, Dietz BM, Pauli GF, van Breemen RB, Bolton JL. Evaluation of estrogenic activity of licorice species in comparison with hops used in botanicals for menopausal symptoms. PLoS One. 2013;8(7):e67947.

[27] Vasudevan K, Sztein JM. Treatment of sperm with extracellular adenosine 5'-triphosphate improves the *in vitro* fertility rate of inbred and genetically modified mice with low fertility. Theriogenology. 2011;76(4):729–736.

[28] Tung NH, Shoyama Y, Wada M, Tanaka H, Improved *in vitro* fertilization ability of mouse dperm caused by the addition of licorice extract to the preincubation medium. The Open Reproductive Sci. J. 2014;6:1–7.

[29] Park D, Yang YH, Choi EK, Yang G, Bae DK, Lee SH, Kim TK, Kyung J, Kim D, Choi KC, Kim YB. Licorice extract increases cyclophosphamide teratogenicity by upregulating the expression of cytochrome P-450 2B mRNA. Birth Defects Res B Dev Reprod Toxicol. 2011;92(6):553–559.

[30] Tanaka H, Baba T. Gene expression in spermiogenesis. Cell Mol Life Sci. 2005;62(3): 344–354.

[31] Fu B, Li H, Wang X, Lee FS, Cui S. Isolation and identification of flavonoids in licorice and a study of their inhibitory effects on tyrosinase. J Agric Food Chem. 2005;53(19): 7408–7414.

[32] Yankep E, Fomum ZT, Bisra D, Dagne E, Hellwig V, Steglich W. *O*-Geranylated isoflavones and a phenylcoumarin from *Millettia griffoniana*. Phytochemistry. 1998;49(8):2521–2523.

[33] Tung HN, Shoyama Y, Wada M, Tanaka H, Two activators of *in vitro* fertilization in mice from licorice. Biochem. Biophys. Res. Commun. 2015;467:447–450.

[34] Carlsen E, Giwercman A, Keiding N, Skakkebaek NE. Evidence for decreasing quality of semen during past 50 years. BMJ. 1992;305(6854):609–613.

Section 3

Action Mechanism of Immunomodulation by Licorice Components

Chapter 8

Isoliquiritigenin: A Unique Component That Attenuates Adipose Tissue Inflammation and Fibrosis by Targeting the Innate Immune Sensors

Yoshinori Nagai, Yasuharu Watanabe,
Hiroe Honda and Kiyoshi Takatsu

Additional information is available at the end of the chapter

http://dx.doi.org/10.5772/66727

Abstract

Recent studies have suggested that pattern recognition receptors, including inflammasomes and TLRs, in the innate immune system recognize various kinds of endogenous ligands and have critical roles in initiating or promoting obesity-associated chronic inflammation. These findings have provided new therapeutic strategies based on regulation of the innate immune system. With the rapid advancement of novel technologies and the increased research on natural products, many new plant-derived extracts and active compounds have been identified to exhibit anti-inflammatory effects. Isoliquiritigenin (ILG) is a flavonoid derived from *Glycyrrhiza uralensis* with a chalcone structure. We have reported that ILG inhibits NLRP3 inflammasome activation resulting in the improvement of diet-induced adipose tissue inflammation and insulin resistance. Furthermore, we have also demonstrated that ILG improves diet-induced fibrosis in adipose tissue by inhibiting TLR4- and Mincle-induced expression of fibrosis-related genes in obese adipose tissue and macrophages. Thus, ILG can suppress two important dysfunctions of obesity, adipose tissue inflammation and fibrosis by targeting innate immune sensors. Here we overview ILG as a potential therapeutic agent for the treatment of obesity-associated diseases. We also summarize anti-inflammatory actions of other constituents of licorice.

Keywords: chronic inflammation, diabetes, inflammasome, innate immunity, metabolic syndrome

1. Introduction

Obesity has become a worldwide health problem because it is strongly associated with metabolic syndromes including type 2 diabetes mellitus (T2DM), atherosclerosis and ischemic heart diseases [1, 2]. Accumulating evidence indicates that chronic low-grade inflammation has a crucial role in the pathogenesis of obesity-associated metabolic dysfunction [3, 4]. The chronic inflammatory alternations are associated with dynamic changes in the composition and function of immune cells in various tissues such as adipose tissue, pancreatic islet, liver, muscle, and hypothalamus [5–7]. A large number of inflammatory immune cells infiltrate into adipose tissue during the course of obesity. M1-like macrophages, an inflammatory type of macrophage, accumulate in adipose tissue and are major sources of inflammatory mediators such as tumor necrosis factor (TNF)-α and IL-6 [8].

The connective fiber content of adipose tissue dramatically increases by the upregulation of collagen expression, which in turn elevates the overall rigidity of adipose tissue and finally leads to fibrosis. The deficiency of collagen 6, a key component of the extracellular matrix in adipose tissue, significantly improves the phenotypes of obese mice, including adipocyte death and adipose tissue inflammation [9]. This implies that alterations in the extracellular matrix in adipose tissue are linked to the development of inflammation. Thus, inflammation and fibrosis are important targets for the treatment of obesity.

An obese state results in an elevation of circulating levels of fatty acids (FAs) and, subsequently, an increase in inflammation of adipose tissue [10]. Adipose macrophages play critical roles in the immune responses through several FA-sensing mechanisms, such as pattern recognition receptors (PRRs). PRRs such as toll-like receptors (TLRs) and nucleotide oligomerization domain (NOD)-like receptors (NLRs) quickly recognize pathogenic agents [11]. It is now becoming even more apparent that these PRRs are not only able to recognize microbial components but also mediate immune responses to endogenous molecules, including those arising in metabolic disorders, such as FAs. These endogenous molecules have been termed danger-associated molecular patterns (DAMPs) and have similar functions as microbial components to activate immune responses [12]. In the obese state, TLR4 may be activated by saturated free FAs, such as palmitic acid, derived from hypertrophied adipocytes as a DAMP and promote adipose tissue inflammation and insulin resistance [13–15]. Inflammasomes are multimeric protein complexes that are crucial for caspase-1, IL-1β, and IL-18 production [16]. The nucleotide-binding domain, leucine-rich repeats containing family, pyrin domain-containing-3 (NLRP3) inflammasome also senses obesity-associated FAs and contributes to obesity-induced inflammation and insulin resistance [17, 18]. Moreover, IL-1β inhibits insulin signaling in the insulin-target organs, including adipose tissue, liver, and skeletal muscle, and also induces dysfunction and cell death of insulin-producing pancreatic β cells [19]. Macrophage-inducible C-type lectin (Mincle) recognizes not only cord factor, a mycobacterial glycolipid, but also SAP130 released from dead cells [20, 21]. Furthermore, Mincle is highly expressed in M1 macrophages in adipose tissue and involved in the induction of adipose tissue fibrosis and insulin resistance during obesity [22, 23].

Plant-derived natural products and their derivatives or synthetic mimics make up a considerable portion of current drugs. These products have played an important role in treating T2DM, especially in Asian countries. We previously reported that glycyrrhizin (GL) and isoliquiritigenin (ILG), components of *Glycyrrhiza uralensis* (*G. uralensis*), inhibit TLR4 signaling at the receptor level on the cell surface, resulting in inhibition of NF-κB and mitogen-activated protein kinases (MAPKs) activation [24]. Furthermore, ILG potently inhibits NLRP3 inflammasome activation independent of its inhibitory action on TLR4 [25]. Our *in vivo* study revealed that ILG attenuated high-fat diet (HFD)-induced adipose tissue inflammation and insulin resistance by inhibiting NLRP3 inflammasome activation in adipose tissue [25]. In addition to inflammation, we recently reported that ILG impacts fibrogenesis in adipose tissue by targeting TLR4 and Mincle activation in macrophages. On the basis of these findings, natural products derived from *G. uralensis* may serve as lead compounds for the development of new anti-T2DM drugs.

This review article highlights the recent discoveries of the anti-inflammatory and anti-fibrotic effects and mechanisms of action of *G. uralensis* components that target PRRs. We will also overview our findings that ILG targets activation of TLR4, NLRP3 inflammasome, and Mincle. We will discuss the roles of innate immunity and potential mechanisms by which it participates in obesity-associated inflammation and fibrosis.

2. PRRs that link with adipose tissue inflammation and fibrosis

2.1. Toll-like receptors

TLRs are transmembrane proteins that recognize conserved structural moieties of microorganisms and for the subsequent induction of pro-inflammatory responses [26]. They directly bind to their ligands and activate the NF-κB and MAPK pathways to induce the production of pro-inflammatory cytokines that are important for evading pathogens. It is widely suggested that TLRs also sense non-microbial endogenous ligands, such as dietary FAs [12]. Activation of TLRs by the endogenous ligands similarly induces pro-inflammatory pathways as microbial ligands in various organs, such as adipose tissue and the liver.

TLR4 is the most important TLR for LPS-mediated inflammatory responses [27]. There is a body of evidence suggesting that TLR4 is an attractive candidate for linking innate immune responses to obesity-associated dysfunction. For example, TLR4 expression is increased in inflammatory macrophages derived from obese adipose tissue [13, 28]. TLR4 KO mice or mice with a loss-of-function mutation in the TLR4 gene are protected from obesity-associated insulin resistance [13, 29]. Furthermore, hematopoietic cell-specific deletion of TLR4 ameliorates HFD-induced hepatic insulin resistance [30]. Intriguingly, saturated FAs released by adipocyte lipolysis can be endogenous TLR4 ligands and activate the NF-κB pathway on macrophages [15]. Another paper reported that resistin derived from adipose tissue directly bound to TLR4 in the hypothalamus and leads to the activation of MAPKs signaling and promoting insulin resistance through MyD88 [31], suggesting that resistin is an endogenous TLR4 ligand, which links hypothalamic inflammation with insulin resistance.

We previously demonstrated that the development of obesity-related inflammation required radioprotective 105 (RP105) rather than TLR4 [32]. RP105 was identified as a first mammalian homologue of Drosophila toll that expressed on B cells [33] and suggested to be involved in LPS-induced B-cell responses. In fact, RP105-deficient mice show reduced LPS-dependent proliferation and CD86 upregulation in B cells, albeit to a lesser extent than TLR4-deficient mice [34, 35]. Among B cell subsets, marginal zone (MZ) B cells express high density of RP105. We have showed that RP105 is indispensable for TLR4-dependent plasma cell differentiation and IgM production in MZ B cells [36]. Additionally, M1 macrophages of murine epididymal white adipose tissue (eWAT) highly express RP105 [32]. This expression is markedly increased by HFD supplementation [32]. Furthermore, HFD-induced obesity, adipose tissue inflammation, and insulin resistance are severely attenuated in RP105 KO mice compared with wild-type (WT) and TLR4 KO mice. In contrast to TLR4, RP105 is not activated by palmitic acid [32]. Our results suggest that ligands and signaling pathways involved in RP105-mediated adipose tissue inflammation do not completely overlap with those utilized by TLR4. Future investigations will determine an endogenous ligand and a signaling pathway of RP105 in adipose tissue.

2.2. NLRP3 inflammasome

Inflammasomes are cytoplasmic receptors and play an important role in the host defense against microbial infection. Activation of NLRP3 inflammasome is regulated by various sterile stimuli, including cholesterol crystals, β-amyloid, palmitic acid, and ceramides. It is generally accepted that two signals are required for NLRP3 inflammasome activation. One is an NF-κB-dependent priming step that induces the transcription of pro-IL-1β and NLRP3. Another is an activation step that induces the activation of caspase-1. Normal activation of NLRP3 inflammasome contributes to host defense, but several studies suggest that excessive activation leads to the development of obesity-associated inflammation.

Islet amyloid polypeptide (IAPP) is deposited in the pancreas and associated with the loss of β cell function in T2DM. The observation of NLRP3-dependent IL-1β production by macrophages in response to IAPP implied a potential role for NLRP3 in promoting IL-1β secretion in T2DM [37]. Interestingly, an anti-diabetic drug glyburide inhibits NLRP3 activation by macrophages in response to IAPP. Direct involvement of NLRP3 in obesity has been confirmed in studies that NLRP3 KO mice fed HFD display reduced caspase-1 activation and pro-IL-1β expression in adipose tissue compared with WT mice [38].

2.3. C-type lectin Mincle

C-type lectin receptors elicit inflammation and innate immune responses through activation of multiple signaling cascades. Mincle recognizes cord factor, a mycobacterial glycolipid, and transduces activation signals by associating with the Fc receptor common γ-chain, which contains immunoreceptor tyrosine-based activation motifs (ITAMs) in the cytoplasmic domain. The phosphorylated ITAM recruits Syk (spleen tyrosine kinase), leading to activation of NF-κB and MAP kinases [39, 40].

The expression level of Mincle is increased by various cellular stresses and stimuli. Mincle expression is upregulated in patients with rheumatoid arthritis and is increased in microglia, neuron, and endothelial cells in the brain after ischemic stroke [41, 42]. Furthermore, Mincle is highly expressed in inflammatory M1 macrophages in adipose tissue and involved in the induction of adipose tissue fibrosis and insulin resistance [22, 23]. These results suggest that

http://dx.doi.org/10.5772/66727

Mincle is involved in the pathogenesis of various inflammation and represents a potential target molecule for the treatment of inflammatory diseases, including rheumatoid arthritis, brain infarction, and T2DM.

3. Natural products that target innate immune system

Chinese herbal formulas with anti-diabetic effects are well developed such that a number of these formulas have commonly been used in diabetic patients since ancient times. The most frequently used 10 Chinese herbs in the period from 2004 to 2009, for the treatment of T2DM, include *Radix Astragali, Rhizome Dioscoreae, Radix Rehnabbiae, Radix Salviae Miltiorrhizae, Radix Puerariae, Rhizoma Coptidis, Fructys Lycii, Poria, Rhizoma Alismatis,* and *Fructus Corni* [43]. However, it is unclear whether these Chinese herbs have as potent anti-inflammatory effects as those of Western anti-diabetic drugs.

Glycyrrhiza plants (licorice) have been used as herbal medicine worldwide for over 4000 years [44]. Several studies have reported that Chinese and Japanese herbal medicines or their components regulate innate immunity. Among *Glycyrrhiza* plants, *G. uralensis* is one of the most used herbal medicines in Asian countries. Various components have been isolated from licorice, for example triterpene saponins, flavonoids, isoflavonoids, and chalcones. Therefore, we have focused on the anti-inflammatory effects of *G. uralensis* and its components on innate immune responses.

3.1. Glycyrrhizin

Glycyrrhizin (GL), a triterpene saponin, is considered to be the major biological active ingredient of *G. uralensis*. It has been reported that GL inhibits LPS-induced TLR4 internalization [45]. Our experiments confirmed that GL suppressed lipid A moiety of LPS-induced IL-6 production in mouse macrophages [24]. Furthermore, GL treatment significantly suppressed the production of inflammatory cytokines, including TNF-α and IL-6, in LPS-injected mice [24]. We further demonstrated that GL attenuated lipid A-mediated activation of NF-κB and MAPKs, including JNK, p38, and ERK. It was suggested that GL might be incorporated into lipid bilayers and suppress the plasma membrane integrity [45]. LPS binds to MD-2 and this triggers homodimerization of the TLR4/MD-2 complex, resulting in the induction of signal transduction [46]. Our data demonstrated that GL inhibited LPS binding to the complex in a dose-dependent manner. Accordingly, LPS-induced TLR4 homodimerization was suppressed by GL stimulation. Moreover, GL inhibited not only LPS- but also TLR9 ligand CpG-DNA-induced inflammatory responses (our unpublished data), as suggested previously [45]. Thus, GL inhibits the activation of multiple TLRs at the plasma membrane by altering membrane integrity.

GL also inhibits the activation of another PRR, NLRP3 inflammasome, induced by various stimuli, including adenosine triphosphate (ATP), monosodium urate (MSU) and nigericin [25]. LPS is a potent inducer of the priming of the NLRP3 inflammasome. However, the inhibitory activity of GL on NLRP3 inflammasome is independent of its effect on TLR4 activation [25]. Intriguingly, activation of another inflammasome, absent in melanoma 2 (AIM2) inflammasome, was suppressed by GL stimulation [25], suggesting that GL inhibits multiple inflammasomes activation. However, a high concentration of GL is required for these inhibitory effects on inflammasomes. Therefore, GL may not be suggested to be a potential therapeutic agent for the treatment of obesity-associated inflammation.

3.2. Isoliquiritigenin

ILG, another component of *G. uralensis*, is a flavonoid with a chalcone structure. It has a wide variety of biological activities, including anti-allergic, anti-tumor growth, and anti-platelet aggregation activity. We recently demonstrated that ILG potently inhibited activation of both TLR4/MD-2 and NLRP3 inflammasome [24, 25]. ILG significantly suppressed LPS-induced production of inflammatory cytokines not only *in vitro* but also *in vivo* [24]. Whereas GL stimulation affects the binding of LPS to TLR4/MD-2, the amount of bound LPS was not decreased by ILG stimulation. However, LPS-induced homotypic interaction of TLR4 was potently inhibited by ILG stimulation in a dose-dependent manner. Additionally, ILG blocked lipid A-induced NF-κB and MAPKs activation [24]. This may be due to the inhibition of TLR4 homodimerization. Beside this, it has been reported that ILG interacts with IKK directly and inhibits its kinase activity [47]. Thus, ILG suppresses TLR4/MD-2-mediated immune responses in multiple steps, at the receptor level and the downstream signaling level (**Figure 1**).

3.2.1. Inhibitory effects of isoliquiritigenin on PRR-mediated adipose tissue inflammation

In addition to the inhibitory effects of ILG on the TLR4/MD-2 complex, we demonstrated that it was highly effective in inhibiting NLRP3 inflammasome activation by various stimuli including ATP, MSU, and nigericin [25]. These responses were suppressed by a low concentration of ILG (10~30 μM). The IC50 for the inhibitory effect of ILG is 0.4936 μM. Furthermore, ILG was more effective in inhibiting NLRP3 inflammasome activation than GL (IC50, 358.9 μM) and parthenolide, a known inhibitor of NLRP3 inflammasome. Contrary to GL, ILG did not inhibit poly(dA:dT)-induced activation of the AIM2 inflammasome. As ILG suppresses NLRP3- but not AIM2-induced formation of ASC pyroptosome, it is unlikely that ASC is a molecular target of ILG. IAPP is a unique polypeptide constituent of amyloid deposited in pancreatic islets [48, 49]. This deposition is associated with disease progression of T2DM and triggers NLRP3 inflammasome activation in islet macrophages [37]. The sulfonylurea drug glyburide inhibits IAPP-induced activation of NLRP3 inflammasome [37]. It is noteworthy that a low concentration of ILG is more effective in inhibiting IAPP-induced activation of NLRP3 inflammasome than that of glyburide [25] (**Figure 1**).

The above observations led us to investigate the inhibitory effects of ILG on TLR4- and NLRP3-associated inflammation in obesity. ILG supplementation remarkably improved obesity, hyperlipidemia, hepatic steatosis, and insulin resistance in HFD-fed wild-type mice [25].

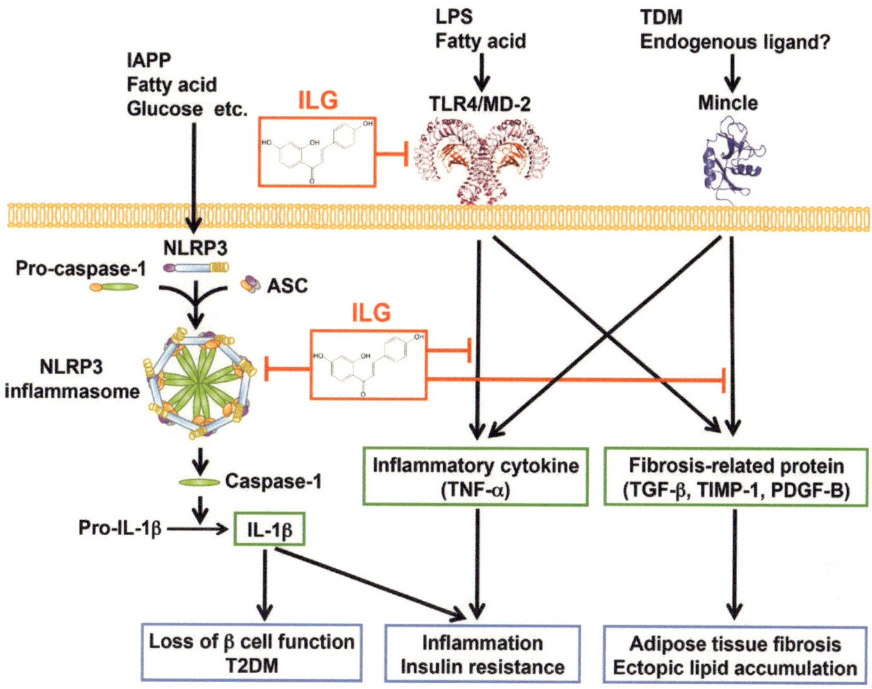

Figure 1. Schematic diagram of ILG-mediated suppression of PRR activation in macrophage. NLRP3 inflammasome is activated by various DAMPs, including IAPP and free FAs. The inflammasomes assemble into oligomeric complex with ASC and activate caspase-1. Activated caspase-1 processes pro-IL-1β into mature IL-1β. ILG potently inhibits IAPP-induced NLRP3 inflammasome activation. The LPS sensor TLR4/MD-2 also recognizes free FAs such as palmitic acid. ILG inhibits TLR4/MD-2-induced inflammation and fibrogenic responses in multiple steps, at the receptor level and the downstream signaling level. Mincle recognizes a mycobacterial glycolipid TDM, also named cord factor. TDM-stimulated inflammatory and fibrogenic responses are attenuated by ILG treatment. Because HFD-induced adipose tissue inflammation and fibrosis are greatly improved in Mincle-deficient mice compared with WT mice, it is suggested that Mincle may recognize an endogenous ligand derived from inflamed tissues, resulting in the induction of inflammation and fibrosis.

Furthermore, ILG supplementation inhibited IL-1β and caspase-1 production in eWAT from wild-type mice fed with HFD for 4 weeks. At this time point, TNF-α production was not increased in eWAT from HFD-fed mice compared with that from normal diet-fed mice. Thus, inflammasome activation occurs in eWAT at an early time point during obesity before TNF-α-associated inflammation.

Because ILG inhibits the priming and activation steps of the inflammasome via TLR4 and NLRP3, respectively, the therapeutic effects of ILG on HFD-induced adipose tissue inflammation and insulin resistance may be attributed to the inhibition of not only NLRP3 but also TLR4 pathways. Indeed, TLR4 is shown to have a critical role in the pathogenesis of obesity-induced inflammation using TLR4-deficient mice [13, 29]. Therefore, ILG is a potential therapeutic agent that targets NLRP3- and TLR4-associated adipose tissue inflammation in obesity.

3.2.2. Inhibitory effects of isoliquiritigenin on PRR-mediated adipose tissue fibrosis

In addition to inflammation, fibrosis may have an important role in adipose tissue dysfunction [9]. Because TLR4 signaling in immune cells has a key role in the development of obesity- and endotoxin-mediated adipose tissue fibrosis [50], we examined whether ILG attenuated TLR4-stimulated expression of fibrosis-related genes in peritoneal macrophages and stromal vascular fraction (SVF) of obese eWAT. Lipid A stimulation increased the expression of fibrosis-related genes, such as TGF-β and TIMP-1 (tissue inhibitor of metalloproteinase-1) in these cells. These increases were significantly attenuated by ILG stimulation (**Figure 1**).

Mincle stimulation is also crucial for fibrogenesis in SVF of obese adipose tissue [22]. The SVF from HFD-fed mice was stimulated with a Mincle ligand trehalose-6,6′-dimycolate (TDM), a mycobacterial cell wall glycolipid [22, 51]. TDM stimulation significantly increased TIMP-1 and PDGF-B mRNA expression in the SVF and these increases were significantly attenuated by ILG stimulation [51] (**Figure 1**).

Finally, we examined whether ILG improved HFD-induced adipose tissue fibrosis. Histological analysis revealed that HFD treatment induced extensive interstitial fibrosis in eWAT, which was markedly suppressed by ILG supplementation (0.5% w/w in HFD) [51]. HFD treatment increased collagen 1, TGF-β, TIMP-1, and PDGF-B mRNA expression in eWAT. These expressions were markedly decreased by ILG supplementation. These results highlight that ILG is a promising therapeutic candidate for HFD-induced adipose tissue fibrosis by suppressing the activation of innate immune sensors.

4. Concluding remarks

It has now become clear that *G. uralensis*-derived components including ILG have a major impact in innate immunity to prevent adipose tissue inflammation and fibrosis. On the other hand, ILG also acts on adipocytes, and consequently suppresses inflammatory changes elicited by macrophage-derived mediators such as TNF-α [51], suggesting that ILG targets multiple cells that constitute adipose tissue. Moreover, activation of various innate immune sensors is affected by ILG stimulation, consequently suppressing adipose tissue inflammation and fibrosis. A better understanding of these mechanisms will be addressed in the near future. With these new findings, we will be enabled to design better therapeutic strategies based on innate immunity through the usage of ILG to combat obesity-associated diseases.

Acknowledgements

We thank all members of our laboratories in the University of Toyama and Toyama Prefectural Institute for Pharmaceutical Research for helpful discussions. The authors sincerely thank Toyama Prefecture for supporting our laboratory.

http://dx.doi.org/10.5772/66727

This work was supported by grants from Grant-in-Aid for Scientific Research from the Japan Society for the Promotion of Science (JSPS) (JSPS KAKENHI Grant Numbers JP16K19532 to Y. W., JP15K08527 to Y.N., JP24390119 to K.T., and JP15K07960 to H.H.), JST, PRESTO (Y.N.), Hokuriku Innovation Cluster for Health Science, MEXT Regional Innovation Cluster Program, Toyama/Ishikawa Region (K.T.), and Hokuriku Life Science Cluster, MEXT Regional Innovation Strategy Support Program (K.T.).

Conflict of interest statement

The authors declare no competing financial interests.

Abbreviations

AIM2	Absent in melanoma 2
ATP	Adenosine triphosphate
DAMP	Danger-associated molecular pattern
eWAT	Epididymal white adipose tissue
FA	Fatty acid
GL	Glycyrrhizin
G. uralensis	*Glycyrrhiza uralensis*
HFD	High-fat diet
IAPP	Islet amyloid polypeptide
ITAM	Immunoreceptor tyrosine-based activation motifs
ILG	Isoliquiritigenin
MAPK	Mitogen-activated protein kinases
Mincle	Macrophage-inducible C-type lectin
MSU	Monosodium urate
MZ	Marginal zone
NLR	NOD-like receptors
NLRP3	Nucleotide-binding domain, leucine-rich repeats containing family, pyrin domain-containing-3
NOD	Nucleotide oligomerization domain
PRR	Pattern recognition receptor
RP105	Radioprotective 105
SVF	Stromal vascular fraction
TDM	Trehalose-6,6′-dimycolate
TIMP-1	Tissue inhibitor of metalloproteinase-1
TLR	Toll-like receptor
TNF	Tumor necrosis factor
T2DM	Type 2 diabetes mellitus
WT	Wild-type

Author details

Yoshinori Nagai[1,2*], Yasuharu Watanabe[1], Hiroe Honda[1,3] and Kiyoshi Takatsu[1,3]

*Address all correspondence to: ynagai@med.u-toyama.ac.jp

1 Department of Immunobiology and Pharmacological Genetics, Graduate School of Medicine and Pharmaceutical Science for Research, University of Toyama, Toyama-shi, Toyama, Japan

2 JST, PRESTO, Saitama, Japan

3 Toyama Prefectural Institute for Pharmaceutical Research, Imizu City, Toyama, Japan

References

[1] G.S. Hotamisligil, Inflammation and metabolic disorders, Nature 444(7121) (2006) 860–7.

[2] S. Schenk, M. Saberi, J.M. Olefsky, Insulin sensitivity: modulation by nutrients and inflammation, J Clin Invest 118(9) (2008) 2992–3002.

[3] N.S. Kalupahana, N. Moustaid-Moussa, K.J. Claycombe, Immunity as a link between obesity and insulin resistance, Mol Aspects Med 33(1) (2012) 26–34.

[4] O. Osborn, J.M. Olefsky, The cellular and signaling networks linking the immune system and metabolism in disease, Nat Med 18(3) (2012) 363–74.

[5] N. Ouchi, J.L. Parker, J.J. Lugus, K. Walsh, Adipokines in inflammation and metabolic disease, Nat Rev Immunol 11(2) (2011) 85–97.

[6] K.K. Ryan, S.C. Woods, R.J. Seeley, Central nervous system mechanisms linking the consumption of palatable high-fat diets to the defense of greater adiposity, Cell Metab 15(2) (2012) 137–49.

[7] C.N. Lumeng, A.R. Saltiel, Inflammatory links between obesity and metabolic disease, J Clin Invest 121(6) (2011) 2111–7.

[8] M. Zeyda, T.M. Stulnig, Adipose tissue macrophages, Immunol Lett 112(2) (2007) 61–7.

[9] T. Khan, E.S. Muise, P. Iyengar, Z.V. Wang, M. Chandalia, N. Abate, B.B. Zhang, P. Bonaldo, S. Chua, P.E. Scherer, Metabolic dysregulation and adipose tissue fibrosis: role of collagen VI, Mol Cell Biol 29(6) (2009) 1575–91.

[10] B.A. Fielding, J. Callow, R.M. Owen, J.S. Samra, D.R. Matthews, K.N. Frayn, Postprandial lipemia: the origin of an early peak studied by specific dietary fatty acid intake during sequential meals, Am J Clin Nutr 63(1) (1996) 36–41.

[11] T. Kawai, S. Akira, The role of pattern-recognition receptors in innate immunity: update on toll-like receptors, Nat Immunol 11(5) (2010) 373–84.

[12] G.Y. Chen, G. Nunez, Sterile inflammation: sensing and reacting to damage, Nat Rev Immunol 10(12) (2010) 826–37.

[13] H. Shi, M.V. Kokoeva, K. Inouye, I. Tzameli, H. Yin, J.S. Flier, TLR4 links innate immunity and fatty acid-induced insulin resistance, J Clin Invest 116(11) (2006) 3015–25.

[14] T. Suganami, J. Nishida, Y. Ogawa, A paracrine loop between adipocytes and macrophages aggravates inflammatory changes: role of free fatty acids and tumor necrosis factor alpha, Arterioscler Thromb Vasc Biol 25(10) (2005) 2062–8.

[15] T. Suganami, K. Tanimoto-Koyama, J. Nishida, M. Itoh, X. Yuan, S. Mizuarai, H. Kotani, S. Yamaoka, K. Miyake, S. Aoe, Y. Kamei, Y. Ogawa, Role of the toll-like receptor 4/NF-kappaB pathway in saturated fatty acid-induced inflammatory changes in the interaction between adipocytes and macrophages, Arterioscler Thromb Vasc Biol 27(1) (2007) 84–91.

[16] E. Latz, T.S. Xiao, A. Stutz, Activation and regulation of the inflammasomes, Nat Rev Immunol 13(6) (2013) 397–411.

[17] H. Wen, D. Gris, Y. Lei, S. Jha, L. Zhang, M.T. Huang, W.J. Brickey, J.P. Ting, Fatty acid-induced NLRP3-ASC inflammasome activation interferes with insulin signaling, Nat Immunol 12(5) (2011) 408–15.

[18] B. Vandanmagsar, Y.H. Youm, A. Ravussin, J.E. Galgani, K. Stadler, R.L. Mynatt, E. Ravussin, J.M. Stephens, V.D. Dixit, The NLRP3 inflammasome instigates obesity-induced inflammation and insulin resistance, Nat Med 17(2) (2011) 179–88.

[19] C.J. Tack, R. Stienstra, L.A. Joosten, M.G. Netea, Inflammation links excess fat to insulin resistance: the role of the interleukin-1 family, Immunol Rev 249(1) (2012) 239–52.

[20] E. Ishikawa, T. Ishikawa, Y.S. Morita, K. Toyonaga, H. Yamada, O. Takeuchi, T. Kinoshita, S. Akira, Y. Yoshikai, S. Yamasaki, Direct recognition of the mycobacterial glycolipid, trehalose dimycolate, by C-type lectin Mincle, J Exp Med 206(13) (2009) 2879–88.

[21] S. Yamasaki, E. Ishikawa, M. Sakuma, H. Hara, K. Ogata, T. Saito, Mincle is an ITAM-coupled activating receptor that senses damaged cells, Nat Immunol 9(10) (2008) 1179–88.

[22] M. Tanaka, K. Ikeda, T. Suganami, C. Komiya, K. Ochi, I. Shirakawa, M. Hamaguchi, S. Nishimura, I. Manabe, T. Matsuda, K. Kimura, H. Inoue, Y. Inagaki, S. Aoe, S. Yamasaki, Y. Ogawa, Macrophage-inducible C-type lectin underlies obesity-induced adipose tissue fibrosis, Nat Commun 5 (2014) 4982.

[23] M. Ichioka, T. Suganami, N. Tsuda, I. Shirakawa, Y. Hirata, N. Satoh-Asahara, Y. Shimoda, M. Tanaka, M. Kim-Saijo, Y. Miyamoto, Y. Kamei, M. Sata, Y. Ogawa, Increased expression of macrophage-inducible C-type lectin in adipose tissue of obese mice and humans, Diabetes 60(3) (2011) 819–26.

[24] H. Honda, Y. Nagai, T. Matsunaga, S. Saitoh, S. Akashi-Takamura, H. Hayashi, I. Fujii, K. Miyake, A. Muraguchi, K. Takatsu, Glycyrrhizin and isoliquiritigenin suppress the LPS sensor toll-like receptor 4/MD-2 complex signaling in a different manner, J Leukoc Biol 91 (6) (2012) 967–76.

[25] H. Honda, Y. Nagai, T. Matsunaga, N. Okamoto, Y. Watanabe, K. Tsuneyama, H. Hayashi, I. Fujii, M. Ikutani, Y. Hirai, A. Muraguchi, K. Takatsu, Isoliquiritigenin is a potent inhibitor of NLRP3 inflammasome activation and diet-induced adipose tissue inflammation, J Leukoc Biol 96(6) (2014) 1087–100.

[26] T. Kawai, S. Akira, The roles of TLRs, RLRs and NLRs in pathogen recognition, Int Immunol 21(4) (2009) 317–37.

[27] K. Hoshino, O. Takeuchi, T. Kawai, H. Sanjo, T. Ogawa, Y. Takeda, K. Takeda, S. Akira, Cutting edge: toll-like receptor 4 (TLR4)-deficient mice are hyporesponsive to lipopolysaccharide: evidence for TLR4 as the Lps gene product, J Immunol 162(7) (1999) 3749–52.

[28] M.T. Nguyen, S. Favelyukis, A.K. Nguyen, D. Reichart, P.A. Scott, A. Jenn, R. Liu-Bryan, C.K. Glass, J.G. Neels, J.M. Olefsky, A subpopulation of macrophages infiltrates hypertrophic adipose tissue and is activated by free fatty acids via toll-like receptors 2 and 4 and JNK-dependent pathways, J Biol Chem 282(48) (2007) 35279–92.

[29] D.M. Tsukumo, M.A. Carvalho-Filho, J.B. Carvalheira, P.O. Prada, S.M. Hirabara, A.A. Schenka, E.P. Araujo, J. Vassallo, R. Curi, L.A. Velloso, M.J. Saad, Loss-of-function mutation in toll-like receptor 4 prevents diet-induced obesity and insulin resistance, Diabetes 56(8) (2007) 1986–98.

[30] M. Saberi, N.B. Woods, C. de Luca, S. Schenk, J.C. Lu, G. Bandyopadhyay, I.M. Verma, J. M. Olefsky, Hematopoietic cell-specific deletion of toll-like receptor 4 ameliorates hepatic and adipose tissue insulin resistance in high-fat-fed mice, Cell Metab 10(5) (2009) 419–29.

[31] Y. Benomar, A. Gertler, P. De Lacy, D. Crepin, H. Ould Hamouda, L. Riffault, M. Taouis, Central resistin overexposure induces insulin resistance through toll-like receptor 4, Diabetes 62(1) (2013) 102-14.

[32] Y. Watanabe, T. Nakamura, S. Ishikawa, S. Fujisaka, I. Usui, K. Tsuneyama, Y. Ichihara, T. Wada, Y. Hirata, T. Suganami, H. Izaki, S. Akira, K. Miyake, H.O. Kanayama, M. Shimabukuro, M. Sata, T. Sasaoka, Y. Ogawa, K. Tobe, K. Takatsu, Y. Nagai, The radioprotective 105/MD-1 complex contributes to diet-induced obesity and adipose tissue inflammation, Diabetes 61(5) (2012) 1199–209.

[33] K. Miyake, Y. Yamashita, M. Ogata, T. Sudo, M. Kimoto, RP105, a novel B cell surface molecule implicated in B cell activation, is a member of the leucine-rich repeat protein family, J Immunol 154(7) (1995) 3333–40.

[34] H. Ogata, I. Su, K. Miyake, Y. Nagai, S. Akashi, I. Mecklenbrauker, K. Rajewsky, M. Kimoto, A. Tarakhovsky, The toll-like receptor protein RP105 regulates lipopolysaccharide signaling in B cells, J Exp Med 192(1) (2000) 23–9.

[35] Y. Nagai, R. Shimazu, H. Ogata, S. Akashi, K. Sudo, H. Yamasaki, S. Hayashi, Y. Iwakura, M. Kimoto, K. Miyake, Requirement for MD-1 in cell surface expression of RP105/CD180 and B-cell responsiveness to lipopolysaccharide, Blood 99(5) (2002) 1699–705.

[36] Y. Nagai, T. Yanagibashi, Y. Watanabe, M. Ikutani, A. Kariyone, S. Ohta, Y. Hirai, M. Kimoto, K. Miyake, K. Takatsu, The RP105/MD-1 complex is indispensable for TLR4/MD-2-dependent proliferation and IgM-secreting plasma cell differentiation of marginal zone B cells, Int Immunol 24(6) (2012) 389–400.

[37] S.L. Masters, A. Dunne, S.L. Subramanian, R.L. Hull, G.M. Tannahill, F.A. Sharp, C. Becker, L. Franchi, E. Yoshihara, Z. Chen, N. Mullooly, L.A. Mielke, J. Harris, R.C. Coll, K.H. Mills, K.H. Mok, P. Newsholme, G. Nunez, J. Yodoi, S.E. Kahn, E.C. Lavelle, L.A. O'Neill, Activation of the NLRP3 inflammasome by islet amyloid polypeptide provides a mechanism for enhanced IL-1beta in type 2 diabetes, Nat Immunol 11(10) (2010) 897–904.

[38] R. Stienstra, J.A. van Diepen, C.J. Tack, M.H. Zaki, F.L. van de Veerdonk, D. Perera, G.A. Neale, G.J. Hooiveld, A. Hijmans, I. Vroegrijk, S. van den Berg, J. Romijn, P.C. Rensen, L. A. Joosten, M.G. Netea, T.D. Kanneganti, Inflammasome is a central player in the induction of obesity and insulin resistance, Proc Natl Acad Sci U S A 108(37) (2011) 15324–9.

[39] M. Cargnello, P.P. Roux, Activation and function of the MAPKs and their substrates, the MAPK-activated protein kinases, Microbiol Mol Biol Rev 75(1) (2011) 50–83.

[40] S. Vallabhapurapu, M. Karin, Regulation and function of NF-kappaB transcription factors in the immune system, Annu Rev Immunol 27 (2009) 693–733.

[41] N. Nakamura, Y. Shimaoka, T. Tougan, H. Onda, D. Okuzaki, H. Zhao, A. Fujimori, N. Yabuta, I. Nagamori, A. Tanigawa, J. Sato, T. Oda, K. Hayashida, R. Suzuki, M. Yukioka, H. Nojima, T. Ochi, Isolation and expression profiling of genes upregulated in bone marrow-derived mononuclear cells of rheumatoid arthritis patients, DNA Res 13(4) (2006) 169–83.

[42] Y. Suzuki, Y. Nakano, K. Mishiro, T. Takagi, K. Tsuruma, M. Nakamura, S. Yoshimura, M. Shimazawa, H. Hara, Involvement of Mincle and Syk in the changes to innate immunity after ischemic stroke, Sci Rep 3 (2013) 3177.

[43] L.W. Qi, E.H. Liu, C. Chu, Y.B. Peng, H.X. Cai, P. Li, Anti-diabetic agents from natural products–an update from 2004 to 2009, Curr Top Med Chem 10(4) (2010) 434–57.

[44] S. Shibata, A drug over the millennia: pharmacognosy, chemistry, and pharmacology of licorice, Yakugaku Zasshi 120(10) (2000) 849–62.

[45] B. Schrofelbauer, J. Raffetseder, M. Hauner, A. Wolkerstorfer, W. Ernst, O.H. Szolar, Glycyrrhizin, the main active compound in liquorice, attenuates pro-inflammatory responses by interfering with membrane-dependent receptor signalling, Biochem J 421 (3) (2009) 473–82.

[46] S. Saitoh, S. Akashi, T. Yamada, N. Tanimura, M. Kobayashi, K. Konno, F. Matsumoto, K. Fukase, S. Kusumoto, Y. Nagai, Y. Kusumoto, A. Kosugi, K. Miyake, Lipid A antagonist, lipid IVa, is distinct from lipid A in interaction with toll-like receptor 4 (TLR4)-MD-2 and ligand-induced TLR4 oligomerization, Int Immunol 16(7) (2004) 961–9.

[47] S. Kumar, A. Sharma, B. Madan, V. Singhal, B. Ghosh, Isoliquiritigenin inhibits IkappaB kinase activity and ROS generation to block TNF-alpha induced expression of cell adhesion molecules on human endothelial cells, Biochem Pharmacol 73(10) (2007) 1602–12.

[48] G.J. Cooper, A.C. Willis, A. Clark, R.C. Turner, R.B. Sim, K.B. Reid, Purification and characterization of a peptide from amyloid-rich pancreases of type 2 diabetic patients, Proc Natl Acad Sci U S A 84(23) (1987) 8628–32.

[49] P. Westermark, C. Wernstedt, E. Wilander, D.W. Hayden, T.D. O'Brien, K.H. Johnson, Amyloid fibrils in human insulinoma and islets of Langerhans of the diabetic cat are derived from a neuropeptide-like protein also present in normal islet cells, Proc Natl Acad Sci U S A 84(11) (1987) 3881–5.

[50] I.K. Vila, P.M. Badin, M.A. Marques, L. Monbrun, C. Lefort, L. Mir, K. Louche, V. Bourlier, B. Roussel, P. Gui, J. Grober, V. Stich, L. Rossmeislova, A. Zakaroff-Girard, A. Bouloumie, N. Viguerie, C. Moro, G. Tavernier, D. Langin, Immune cell toll-like receptor 4 mediates the development of obesity- and endotoxemia-associated adipose tissue fibrosis, Cell Rep 7(4) (2014) 1116–29.

[51] Y. Watanabe, Y. Nagai, H. Honda, N. Okamoto, S. Yamamoto, T. Hamashima, Y. Ishii, M. Tanaka, T. Suganami, M. Sasahara, K. Miyake, K. Takatsu, Isoliquiritigenin attenuates adipose tissue inflammation in vitro and adipose tissue fibrosis through inhibition of innate immune responses in mice, Sci Rep 6 (2016) 23097.

Chapter 9

Novel Mechanism Supporting Therapeutic Effects of Glycyrrhizin in Acute or Chronic Hepatitis

Noriyuki Kuroda and Tetsuji Sato

Additional information is available at the end of the chapter

http://dx.doi.org/10.5772/67078

Abstract

Glycyrrhizin (GL) isolated from the roots of licorice plant (*Glycyrrhiza glabra* L.) has been traditionally used for treating peptic ulcer, hepatitis, and pulmonary bronchitis. In addition to the protective effects of GL against liver injury or cancer proliferation by the membrane stabilization or via progesterone-receptor membrane component 1 (PGRMC1), the present chapter reports its new therapeutic mechanism through high-mobility group protein 1 (HMGB1) to which GL directly binds. In this study, we evaluated inflammation-promoting activity of HMGB1 and blockade of extracellular release of HMGB1 by GL in lipopolysaccharide (LPS)/D-galactosamine (GalN)-triggered mouse liver injury. In this experimental hepatitis model, apoptotic response of hepatocytes through the binding of HMGB1 protein to Glutathione transferase omega 1 (*Gsto1*), an apoptosis-associated gene, promoter region is caused, serum AST and ALT activities significantly increased, and GL-treatment prevented the apoptosis and inflammatory infiltrates induced with LPS/GalN-injection by disturbing the binding of HMGB1 protein to *Gsto1* promoter sequence. Analysis with chromatin immunoprecipitation (ChIP)-assay revealed inhibiting the binding of HMGB1 protein to *Gsto1* by the binding of GL to HMGB1.

Keywords: glycyrrhizin, liver injury, PAMPs, DAMPs, HMGB1

1. Introduction

Glycyrrhizin (GL), a triterpenoid glycoside isolated from the roots of licorice plant (*Glycyrrhiza glabra* L.), has been traditionally used for treating peptic ulcer, hepatitis, and pulmonary bronchitis. Various pharmacological effects of GL are well known, such as anti-inflammatory [1, 2], anti-allergic [3], and hepatoprotective activity [4–6]. In Japan, Stronger Neo-Minophagen C, the active ingredient of which is GL, has been used as a treatment for over 25 years for patients with chronic hepatitis. Intravenous administration of GL decreases serum alanine aminotransferase (ALT) and aspartate aminotransferase (AST) levels in patients with chronic hepatitis [7, 8]. The well-defined model of hepatic injury induced by the injection of lipopolysaccharide (LPS)/D-galactosamine (GalN) has been widely used in studies of the mechanisms of human hepatitis. GalN is an aminosugar selectively metabolized by hepatocytes, which induces a depletion of the uridine triphosphate pool and thereby an inhibition of macromolecule (RNA, protein, and glycogen) synthesis in the liver [9]. Combination of LPS and GalN causes specifically hepatic failure in rodent [10]. Under the stimulation by LPS, liver macrophages secrete various pro-inflammatory cytokines including tumor necrosis factor (TNF)-α which is a terminal mediator for apoptosis, subsequently leading to hepatic necrosis [11–14]. The hepatic lesion in this model resembles that of human hepatitis since the up-regulation of TNF-α level and hepatic apoptosis have been reported as pathogenic symptoms in human hepatitis. GL, an aqueous extract of licorice root, has been used for the treatment of chronic hepatitis to reduce the liver inflammation [15–17], but its effects on acute hepatic injury have been unclear. A recent report showed that Y-40138, a synthetic compound, inhibits liver injury evoked by LPS/GalN through the suppression of TNF-α and monocyte chemoattractant protein-1 and the augmentation of IL-10 [18]. GL prevents anti-Fas antibody-induced mouse liver injury but has no effect on the upregulation of TNF-α mRNA expression in the liver [6]. In our previous study [19], we reported that levels of serum of cytokines such as TNF-α, interleukin (IL)-6, IL-10, IL-12, and IL-18 as well as those of serum ALT significantly increased after administration of LPS/GalN. GL had no effect on the production of TNF-α, IL-6, IL-10, and IL-12, whereas it significantly inhibited the increase in ALT levels and IL-18 production. We have so far indicated that the inhibitory effect of GL is different from that of inhibitor for TNF-α production, such as Y-40138 [18] and bicyclol, a new synthetic anti-hepatitis drug [20].

High-mobility group proteins (HMGBs) possess a unique DNA-binding domain that is subject to transcriptional regulation [21]. One of these proteins, HMGB1 (amphoterin), can be secreted into the extracellular milieu as a late-acting mediator of LPS-induced or sepsis-induced lethality in mice [22]. Although HMGB1 is a non-histone nuclear protein, it is passively released from necrotic cells [23] or actively secreted from stress-received cells such as monocytes/macrophages as an inflammatory cytokine in response to endotoxin, tumor necrosis factor (TNF)-α, or interleukin (IL)-1β [22, 24–26]. HMGB1, which was released into the intravascular area, has great potential as a local inflammatory activator through intensifying the release of cytokines and chemokines from stimulated cells [27] and interact with endothelial cells by up-regulating surface receptors and causing the secretion of soluble pro-inflammatory mediators [28]. Extracellular HMGB1 works properly as a damage-associated molecular patterns (DAMPs) molecule and increases powers of pro-inflammatory signaling paths by activating pattern recognition receptors (PRRs) including toll-like receptor 4 (TLR4) and/or the receptor for advanced glycation end-products (RAGE) [25, 29]. Increasing evidence suggests that HMGB1 may also operate so as to assist the progress of the recognition of other immune co-activators such as LPS, DNA, and IL-1 by being excessively desirous of the binding to these molecules [30–32]. However, the mechanisms by which GL inhibits inflammation induced with pathogen-associated molecular patterns (PAMPs) such as LPS or endogenous DAMPs such as HMGB1 have not been clearly revealed.

Previous results have suggested that glycyrrhizin (GL) and glycyrrhetinic acid (GA) exert their protective effects by the membrane stabilization which results in inhibiting the prolongation of oxidative stress [33]. Furthermore, progesterone-receptor membrane component 1 (PGRMC1) was proposed as a new target protein for GL. PGRMC1 is a haem-containing protein that inter-

http://dx.doi.org/10.5772/67078

acts with epidermal growth factor (FGFR) and cytochrome P450 to regulate cancer proliferation and chemoresistance [34]. GL is thought to reduce cancer proliferation via PGRMC1. On the other hand, a research work utilizing nuclear magnetic resonance (NMR) and fluorescence methods revealed the supplementary mechanism by which GL directly binds to HMGB1 and suppresses the HMGB1 chemoattractant and mitogenic activities [35]. Recent studies, furthermore, have reported that GL reduces inflammatory infiltrates by inhibiting the cellular proliferation and migration, and formation of blood vessels induced by HMGB1 [36]. In this chapter, we evaluated the underlying new mechanism supporting various pharmacological effects of GL on the basis of upcoming data of our experiment on hepatitis induced by an injection of LPS/GalN.

2. Results and discussion

In the present study, we explored inflammation-promoting activity of HMGB1 and blockade of extracellular release of HMGB1 by GL in LPS/GalN-triggered mouse liver injury. Male BALB/c mice were intravenously injected with LPS/GalN. At 1–10 h after LPS/GalN treatment, mice were anesthetized to collect blood by heart puncture, and serum transaminase and HMGB1 were evaluated. Intraperitoneal administration of GL was performed 30 min before treatment. Effects of GL on liver damage were examined 8 h after stimulation with endotoxin. The injection of LPS/GalN significantly increases serum AST and ALT activities as compared with controls. The enhancement of AST and ALT levels is significantly suppressed by an intraperitoneal administration of GL (**Figure 1**; [19, 37, 38]). Administration of LPS/GalN precipitate tissue injury associated with time-dependent alteration in HMGB1 serum levels. Immunohistochemistry with antibodies to HMGB1 reveals a distinct nuclear expression in the hepatocytes of control mice. Immunoreactivity to HMGB1 begins to be suppressed in the nuclei 6 h after administration of LPS/GalN. At 8 h nuclear immunoreactive products are remarkably reduced and extracellular HMGB1 expression is found exclusively in the pericentral foci. Double-immunofluorescence staining for HMGB1/F4/80 or HMGB1/CD11c demonstrates that some cell populations of $F4/80^+$ and $CD11c^+$ cells located in the inflammatory foci are immunolabeled simultaneously with HMGB1 8 h after stimulation with LPS/GalN [39]. The GL-treatment significantly reduces the serum levels of ALT, AST, and HMGB1 besides the strong inhibition of inflammatory tissue damage, and cytoplasmic and extracellular immunoreactive-response to both the HMGB1 and acetylated-lysine. The acetylation of HMGB1 is physiologically involved in regulating HMGB1 DNA binding properties along with the subcellular location. The lysine residues of HMGB1 between 27 and 43 represent functional nuclear localizing signals. An administration of GL brings about a significant decrease in the number of apoptotic hepatocytes labeled with TUNEL-method. On the basis of these results, we have identified an apoptosis-associated gene, Glutathione transferase omega 1 (*Gsto1*), using microarray analysis and real-time PCR (**Figure 2**). In addition, the chromatin immunoprecipitation (ChIP)-assay have revealed the binding of HMGB1 protein to *Gsto1* promoter sequence and the remarkable decrease in the volume of bound HMGB1 protein by administration of GL (**Figure 3**). Our findings claim that GL treatment might prevent the apoptosis and inflammatory infiltrate caused with LPS/GalN-treatment by disturbing the binding of HMGB1 protein to *Gsto1* promoter sequence. We provide *in vivo* evidence showing that HMGB1 is involved in the apoptosis of hepatocytes caused by LPS/GalN-treatment and administration of GL significantly improves hepatic injury, in parallel with suppression of exaggerated apoptotic cell death and enhanced expression of regeneration mediator. Several recent investigations including our research [40] have reported that GL may protect against liver injury by reducing the expression of HMGB1, a mediator of inflammation [41, 42]. The induction of liver injury in mice by LPS/GalN represents a promising animal model for elucidating the mechanism of clinical dysfunction and for evaluating the efficacy of hepatoprotectives. The liver injury induced by LPS has been reported to be abrogated by treatment with anti-TNF-α mAb or p55 TNF receptors in mice [43–45]. TNF-α can induces apoptosis of hepatocytes at an early stage in LPS/GalN-induced liver injury, and neutrophil transmigration can represent a critical step leading to necrosis of hepatocytes at a later stage [46, 47]. In our study [19], the serum levels of TNF-α were markedly increased 0.5–1 h after LPS/GalN-treatment. Treatment with anti-TNF-α antibody reduced the elevated ALT level by LPS/GalN. Thus, it appears that TNF-α plays an important role in the pathogenesis of this model. There is evidence for the cytoprotection by IL-6 of liver injury induced by LPS [48]. In addition, both endogenous and exogenous IL-10 protect against LPS/GalN-induced liver injury [49]. Others have reported that at a 2-h timepoint, IL-12 is increased in plasma of mice treated with LPS/GalN [13]. We have confirmed that the serum levels of IL-6, IL-10, and IL-12 can reach a maximum by 2 h after LPS/GalN treatment [19]. GL had no effect on the production of TNF-α, IL-6, IL-10, and IL-12 in the same model mice, whereas it significantly inhibited increase in ALT levels.

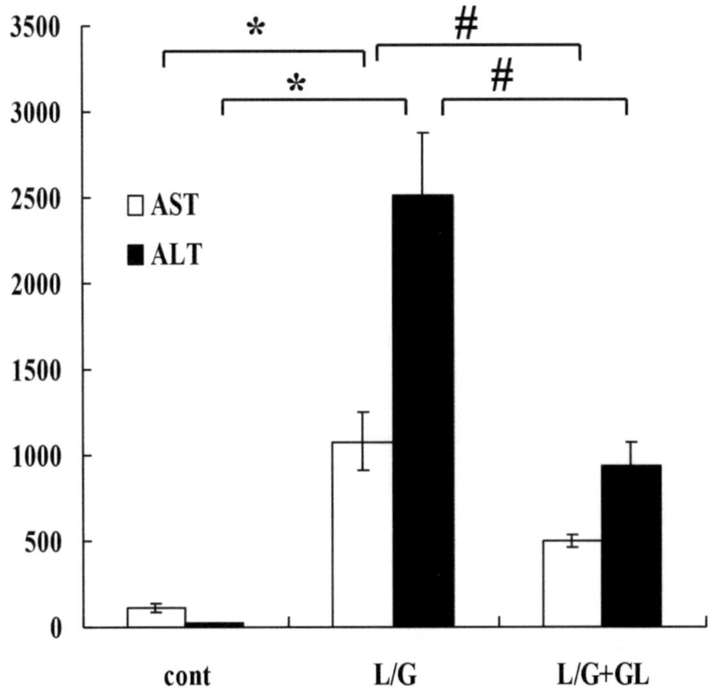

Figure 1. The effect of GL on serum AST and ALT levels at 8 h after administration of LPS/D-GalN. Increased serum AST and ALT levels are significantly inhibited by combined treatment with LPS/D-GalN + GL (L/G + GL) compared with mice treated with L/G. *Significant difference compared with 0 h or control ($P < 0.05$); #Significant difference between L/G and L/G + GL ($P < 0.05$); each value represents the mean ± SEM of six mice (Cited from Ref. [38]).

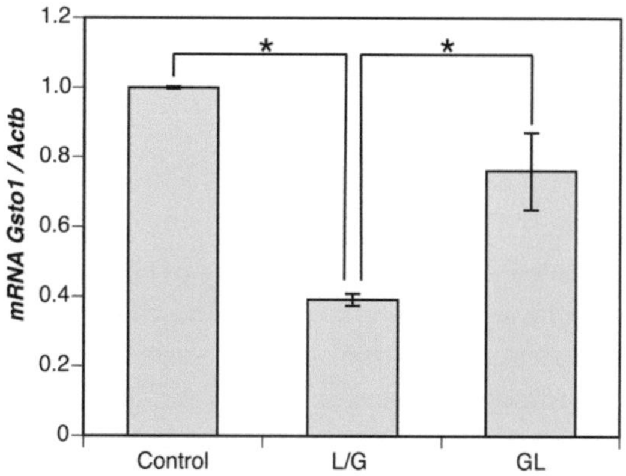

Figure 2. mRNA expression of *Gsto1* gene involved in apoptosis by LPS/GalN-treatment. After an injection of LPS/GalN, the expression level of *Gsto1* mRNAs is significantly decreased. The expression level of *Gsto1* mRNA is significantly recovered by administration of GL. *Significant difference between two groups (Control versus LPS/GalN or LPS/GalN versus GL + LPS/GalN) approved ($P < 0.05$). L/G: LPS/GalN, GL: GL + LPS/GalN (Cited from Ref. [40]).

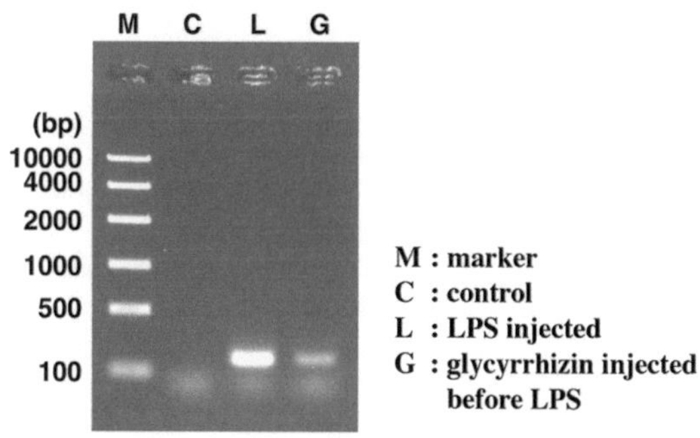

Figure 3. Analysis of HMGB1-binding to *Gsto1* with chromatin immunoprecipitation (ChIP)-assay. Hmgb1 protein intensely binds to *Gsto1* promoter sequence in LPS/GalN-induced liver injury and an administration of GL remarkably inhibits the binding of Hmgb1 to *Gsto1* promoter sequence. M: marker, C: control, L: LPS/GalN, G: GL + LPS/GalN (Cited from Ref. [40]).

HMGB1 is a multifunctional protein: the earliest studies reported it as a nonhistone DNA-binding nuclear protein. HMGB1 binds to DNA in a sequence-independent manner and changes the structure of DNA so as to assist the progress of transcription, replication, and repair [50, 51]. These functions are essential for survival, as HMGB1-deficient mice die of hypoglycemia within 24 h after birth [52]. Recent researches have identified HMGB1 as a new inflammatory factor and a late mediator of endotoxin lethality in mice [53]. Extracellularly released HMGB1 mobilizes a great number of various physiological reactions in different cell types [54]. HMGB1 may be released both through active secretion from various cells, including activated monocytes/macrophages [22], neutrophils [55], and endothelial cells [56], and passively from necrotic or damaged cells [23]. HMGB1 is released as a danger signal from damaged cells [24]. Even when cellular integrity is maintained, hepatocyte HMGB1 expression increases markedly after noxious stimuli [13, 24]. In our experiment, immunohistochemistry revealed

HMGB1 overexpression was found predominantly in the inflammatory foci located close to the central veins, that is, in areas most susceptible to LPS/GalN-treatment.

3. Conclusion

Apoptotic response of hepatocytes through the binding of HMGB1 protein to *Gsto1* promoter region is caused in this experimental hepatitis model and GL-treatment prevents the apoptosis and inflammatory infiltrates caused with LPS/GalN-injection by disturbing the binding of HMGB1 protein to *Gsto1* promoter sequence. The present findings claim a new mechanism supporting therapeutic effects of GL in hepatitis (**Figure 4**).

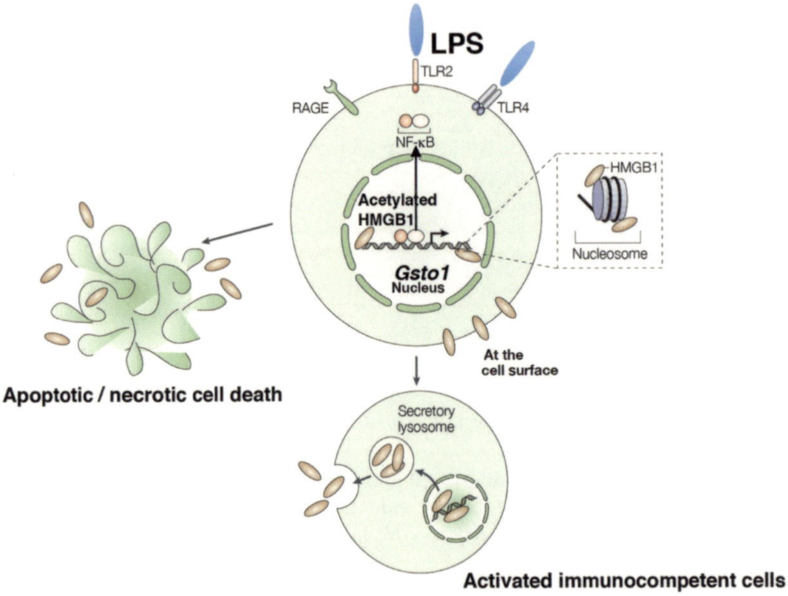

Figure 4. Action point of acetylated HMGB1. An administration of GL suppresses apoptotic cell death through inhibiting the binding of Hmgb1 to *Gsto1* (Scheme modified from Nature Reviews Immunology 2005:5:334).

Author details

Noriyuki Kuroda and Tetsuji Sato*

*Address all correspondence to: sato-t@tsurumi-u.ac.jp

Department of Anatomy, Tissue, and Cell Biology, School of Dental Medicine, Tsurumi University, Yokohama, Japan

References

[1] Ohuchi K, Kamada Y, Levine L, Tsurufuji S. Glycyrrhizin inhibits prostaglandin E2 production by activated peritoneal macrophages from rats. Prostaglandins and Medicine. 1981;7:457–463.

[2] Okimasu E, Moromizato Y, Watanabe S, Sasaki J, Shiraishi N, Morimoto YM, Miyahara M, Utsumi K. Inhibition of phospholipase A2 and platelet aggregation by glycyrrhizin, an antiinflammation drug. Acta Medica Okayama. 1983;**37**:385–391.

[3] Kuroyanagi T, Saito M. Effect of prednisolone and glycyrrhizin on passive transfer in experimental allergic encephalomyelitis. Arerugi. 1966;**15**:67–74.

[4] Nose M, Ito M, Kamimura K, Shimizu M, Ogihara Y. A comparison of the antihepatotoxic activity between glycyrrhizin and glycyrrhetinic acid. Planta Medica. 1994;**60**:136–139.

[5] Okamoto T, Kanda T. Glycyrrhizin protects mice from concanavalin A-induced hepatitis without affecting cytokine expression. International Journal of Molecular Medicine. 1999;**4**:149–152.

[6] Okamoto T. The protective effect of glycyrrhizin on anti-Fas antibody-induced hepatitis in mice. European Journal of Pharmacology. 2000;**387**:229–232.

[7] Arase Y, Ikeda K, Murashima N, Chayama K, Tsubota A, Koida I, Suzuki Y, Saitoh S, Kobayashi M, Kumada H. The long term efficacy and glycyrrhizin in chronic hepatitis C patients. Cancer. 1997;**79**:1494–1500.

[8] Ikeda K, Arase Y, Kobayashi M, Saitoh S, Someya T, Hosokawa T, Senzaki H, Akuta N, Suzuki Y, Suzuki F, Kumada H. A long-term glycyrrhizin injection therapy reduces hepatocellular carcinogenesis rate in patients with interferon-resistant active chronic hepatitis C: a cohort study of 1249 patients. Digestive Diseases and Sciences. 2006;**51**:603–609.

[9] Decker K, Keppler D. Galactosamine hepatitis: key role of the nucleotide deficiency period in the pathogenesis of cell injury and cell death. Reviews of Physiology, Biochemistry and Pharmacology. 1974;**71**:77–106.

[10] Galanos C, Freudenberg MA, Reutter W. Galactosamine-induced sensitization to the lethal effects of endotoxin. Proceedings of the National Academy of Sciences of the United States of America. 1979;**76**:5939–5943.

[11] Tiegs G, Wolter M, Wendel A. Tumor necrosis factor is a terminal mediator in galactosamine/endotoxin-induced hepatitis in mice. Biochemical Pharmacology. 1989; **38**:627–631.

[12] Leist M, Gantner F, Bohlinger I, Toegs G, Gertmann PG, Wendel A. Tumor necrosis factor-induced hepatocyte apoptosis precedes liver failure in experimental murine shock models. The American Journal of Pathology. 1995;**146**:1220–1234.

[13] Sass G, Heinlein S, Agli A, Bang R, Schumann J, Tiegs G. Cytokine expression in three mouse model of experimental hepatitis. Cytokine. 2002;**19**:115–120.

[14] Morikawa A, Sugiyama T, Kato Y, Koide N, Jiang G, Takahashi K, Tamada Y, Yokochi T. Apoptotic cell death in the response of D-galactosamine-sensitized mice to lipopolysaccharide as an experimental endotoxic shock model. Infection and Immunity. 1996, **64**:734–738.

[15] Takahara T, Watanabe A, Shiraki K. Effects of glycyrrhizin on hepatitis B surface antigen: a biochemical and morphological study. Journal of Hepatology. 1994;**21**:601–609.

[16] Ito A, Hayashi N, Katayama K, Hagiwara H, Kasahara A, Kashiwagi T, Yoshihara H, Fusamoto H, Kamada T. Effect of glycyrrhizin on viral replication and quasispecies in patients with type C chronic hepatitis. International Hepatology Communications. 1997;**6**:233–238.

[17] Yoshikawa M, Matsui Y, Kawamoto H, Umemoto N, Oku K, Koizumi M, Yamao J, Kuriyama S, Nakano H, Hozumi N, Ishizaka S, Fukui H. Effects of glycyrrhizin on immune-mediated cytotoxicity. Journal of Gastroenterology and Hepatology. 1997; **12**:243–248.

[18] Fukuda T, Mogami A, Tanaka H, Yoshikawa T, Hisadome M, Komatsu H. Y-40138, a multiple cytokine production modulator, protects against D-galactosamine and lipopolysaccharide-induced hepatitis. Life Sciences. 2006;**79**:822–827.

[19] Yoshida T, Abe K, Ikeda T, Matsushita T, Wake K, Sato T, Sato To, Inoue H. Inhibitory effect of glycyrrhizin on lipopolysaccharide and D-galactosamine-induced mouse liver injury. European Journal of Pharmacology. 2007;**576**:136–142.

[20] Wang H, Li Y. Protective effect of bicyclol on acute hepatic failure induced by lipopolysaccharide and D-galactosamine in mice. European Journal of Pharmacology. 2006;**534**:194–201.

[21] Bustin M, Hopkins RB, Isenberg I. Immunological relatedness of high mobility group chromosomal proteins from calf thymus. The Journal of Biological Chemistry. 1978;**253**:1694–1699.

[22] Wang H, Bloom O, Zhang M, Vishnubhakat JM, Ombrellino M, Che JH, Ivanova S, Borovikova L, Manogure LR, Faist E, Abraham E, Andersson U, Molina PR, Abumrad NN, Sama A, Tracey KJ. HMG-1 as a late mediator of endotoxin lethality in mice. Science. 1999;**285**:248–251.

[23] Scaffidi P, Misteli T, Bianchi ME. Release of chromatin protein HMGB1 by necrotic cells triggers inflammation. Nature. 2002;**418**:191–195.

[24] Tsung A, Sahai R, Tanaka H, Nakao A, Fink MP, Lotze MT, Yang H, Li J, Tracey KJ, Geller DA, Billiar TR. The nuclear factor HMGB1 mediates hepatic injury after murine liver ischemia-reperfusion. The Journal of Experimental Medicine. 2005;**201**:1135–1143.

[25] Tsung A, Klune JR, Zhang X, Jeyabalan G, Cao Z, Peng X, Stolz DB, Geller DA, Rosengart MR, Billiar TR. HMGB1 release induced by liver ischemia involves toll-like receptor 4-dependent reactive oxygen species production and calcium-mediated signaling. The Journal of Experimental Medicine. 2007;**204**:2913–2923.

[26] Ilmakunnas M, Tukiainen A, Rauvala H, Arola J, Nordin A, Mäkisalo H, Höckerstedt K, Isoniemi H. High mobility group box 1 protein as a marker of hepatocellular injury in human liver transplantation. Liver Transplantation. 2008;**14**:1517–1525.

[27] Andersson U, Wang H, Palmblad K, Aveberger AC, Bloom O, Erlandsson-Harris H, Janson A, Kokkola R, Zhang M, Yang H, Tracey KJ. High mobility group 1 protein (HMG-1) stimulates proinflammatory cytokine synthesis in human monocytes. The Journal of Experimental Medicine. 2000;**192**:565–570.

[28] Fiuza C, Bustin M, Talwar S, Tropea M, Gerstenberger E, Shelhamer JH, Suffredini AF. Inflammation-promoting activity of HMGB1 on human microvascular endothelial cells. Blood. 2003;**101**:2652–2660.

[29] Hori O, Brett J, Slattery T, Cao R, Zhang J, Chen X, Nagashima M, Lundh ER, Vijay S, Nitecki D, Morsert J, Stern D, Schmidt AM. The receptor for advanced glycation end products (RAGE) is a cellular binding site for amphoterin. The Journal of Biological Chemistry. 1995;**270**:25752–25761.

[30] Ivanov S, Dragoi A-M, Wang X, Dallacosta C, Louten J, Musco G, Sitia G, Yap GS, Wan Y, Biron CA, Bianchi ME, Wang H, Chu W-M. A novel role for HMGB1 in TLR9-mediated inflammatory responses to CpG-DNA. Blood. 2007;**110**:1970–1981.

[31] Tian J, Avalos AM, Mao S-Y, Chen B, Senthil K, Wu H, Parroche P, Drabic S, Golenbock D, Sirois C, Hua J, An LL, Audoly L, Rosa GL, Bierhaus A, Naworth P, Marshak-Rothstein A, Crow MK, Fitzgerald KA, Latz E, Kiener RA, Coele AJ. Toll-like receptor 9-dependent activation by DNA-containing immune complexes is mediated by HMGB1 and RAGE. Nature Immunology. 2007;**8**:487–496.

[32] Sha Y, Zmijewski J, Xu Z, Abraham E. HMGB1 develops enhanced proinflammatory activity by binding to cytokines. The Journal of Immunology. 2008;**180**:2531–2537.

[33] Takayama F, Egashira T, Yamanaka Y. Effects of glycyrrhizin and glycyrrhetinic acid on damage to isolated hepatocytes by transient exposure to *tert*-butyl hydroperoxide. Japanese Pharmacology and Therapeutics. 2000;**28**:763–770.

[34] Kabe Y, Nakane T, Koike I, Yamamoto T, Sugiura Y, Harada E, Sugase K, Shimamura T, Ohmura M, Muraoka K, Yamamoto A, Uchida T, Iwata S, Yamaguchi Y, Krayukhina E, Nada M, Handa H, Ishimori K, Uchiyama S, Kobayashi T, Suematsu M. Haem-dependent dimerization of PGRMC1/Sigma-2 receptor facilitates cancer proliferation and chemoresistance. Nature Communications. 2016;**7**:11030. doi: 10.1038/ncomms11030

[35] Mollica L, Marchis FD, Spitaleri A, Dallacosta C, Pennacchini D, Zamai M, Agresti A, Trisciuoglio L, Musco G, Bianchi ME. Glycyrrhizin binds to high-mobility group box 1 protein and inhibits its cytokine activities. Chemistry & Biology. 2007;**14**:431–441.

[36] Smolarczyk R, Cichoñ T, Matuszczak S, Mitrus I, Lesiak M, Kobusiñska M, Kamysz W, Jarosz M, Sieroñ A, Szala S. The role of glycyrrhizin, an inhibitor of HMGB1 protein, in anticancer therapy. Archivum Immunologiae et Therapiae Experimentalis. 2012;**60**:391–399.

[37] Abe K, Ikeda T, Wake K, Sato T, Sato T, Inoue H. Glycyrrhizin prevents lipopolysacchararide/D-galactosamine-induced liver injury through down-regulation of matrix metalloproteinase-9 in mice. Journal of Pharmacy and Pharmacology. 2008;**60**:91–97.

[38] Ikeda T, Abe K, Kuroda N, Kida Y, Inoue H, Wake K, Morito M, Sato T. The inhibition of apoptosis by glycyrrhizin in hepatic injury induced by injection of lipopolysaccharide/D-garactosamine in mice. Archives of Histology and Cytology. 2008;**71**:163–178.

[39] Sato T, Yamamoto H, Sasaki C, Wake K. Maturation of rat dendritic cells during intrahepatic translocation evaluated using monoclonal antibodies and electron microscopy. Cell and Tissue Research. 1998;**294**:503–514.

[40] Kuroda N, Inoue K, Ikeda T, Hara Y, Wake K, Sato T. Apoptotic response through a high mobility box 1 protein-dependent mechanism in LPS/GalN-induced mouse liver failure and glycyrrhizin-mediated inhibition. PLoS One. 2014;**9**:e92884. doi: 10.1371/jounal.pone.0092884

[41] Mabuchi A, Wake K, Marlini M, Watanabe H, Wheatley AM. Protection by glycyrrhizin against warm ischemia-reperfusion-induced cellular injury and derangement of the microcirculatory blood flow in the rat liver. Microcirculation. 2009;**16**:364–376. doi: 10.1080/10739680902796917

[42] Ogiku M, Kono H, Hara M, Tsuchiya M, Fujii H. Glycyrrhizin prevents liver injury by inhibition of high-mobility group box 1 production by Kupffer cells after ischemia-reperfusion in rats. Journal of Pharmacology and Experimental Therapeutics. 2011;**339**:93–98. doi: 10.1124/jpet.111.182592

[43] Beutler B, Milsark IS, Cerami AC. Passive immunization against cachectin/tumor necrosis factor protects mice from lethal effect of endotoxin. Science. 1985;**229**:869–871.

[44] Tracy KJ, Fong Y, Hesse DG, Manogue KR, Lee AT, Kuo GC, Lowry SF, Cerami A. Anti-cachectin/TNF monoclonal antibodies prevent septic shock during lethal bacteraemia. Nature. 1987;**330**:662–664.

[45] Lesslauer W, Tabuchi H, Gentz R, Brockhaus, M, Schlaeger EJ, Grau G, Piguet PF, Pointaire P, Vassalli P, Loetscher H. Recombinant soluble tumor necrosis factor receptor proteins protect mice from lipopolysaccharide-induced lethality. European Journal of Immunology. 1991;**21**:2883–2886.

[46] Tiegs G. Immunotoxicology of host-response-mediated experimental liver injury. Journal of Hepatology. 1994;**21**:890–903.

[47] Chosay, JS, Essani NA, Dunn CJ, Jaeschke H. Neutrophil margination and extravasation in sinusoids and venules of liver during endotoxin-induced injury. The American Journal of Physiology. 1997;**272**(5 pt 1):G1195–G1200.

[48] Inoue K, Takano H, Shimada A, Morita T, Yanagisawa R, Sakurai M, Sato M, Yoshino S, Yoshikawa T. Cytoprotection by interleukin-6 against liver injury induced by lipopolysaccharide. International Journal of Molecular Sciences. 2005;**15**:221–224.

[49] Louis H, Moine OL, Peny MO, Gulbis B, Nisol F, Goldman M, Deviere J. Hepatoprotevtive role of interleukin 10 in galactosamine/lipopolysaccharide mouse liver injury. Gastroenterology. 1997;**112**:935–942.

[50] Johns EW. Studies on histone. 8. A degradation product of lysine-rich histone. Biochemical Journal. 1964;**93**:161–163.

[51] Bustin M. Regulation of DNA-dependent activities by the functional motifs of the high-mobility-group chromosomal proteins. Molecular and Cellular Biology. 1999;**19**:5237–5246.

[52] Calogero S, Grassi F, Aguzzi A, Voigtländer T, Ferrier P, Ferrari S, Bianchi ME. The lack of chromosomal protein Hmg1 does not disrupt cell growth but causes lethal hypoglycaemia in newborn mice. Nature Genetics. 1999;**22**:276–280.

[53] Wang Y, Liu J, Wu Y, Luo W, Lin SH, Lin H, Hawk N, Sun T, Guo JQ, Estrov Z, Talpaz M, Champlin R, Arlinghaus RB: Expression of a truncated first exon BCR sequence in chronic myelogenous leukemia cells blocks cell growth and induces cell death. Cancer Research. 2001;**61**:4112–4121.

[54] Yang H, Wang H, Czura CJ, Tracey KJ. The cytokine activity of HMGB1. Journal of Leukocyte Biology. 2005;**78**:1–8.

[55] Ito I, Fukazawa J, Yoshida M. Post-translational methylation of high mobility group box 1 (HMGB1) causes its cytoplasmic localization in neutrophils. The Journal of Biological Chemistry. 2007;**282**:16336–16344.

[56] Mullins GE, Sunden-Cullberg J, Johansson AS, Rouhiainen A, Erlandsson-Harris H, Yang H, Tracey KJ, Rauvala H, Palmblad J, Andersson J, Treutiger CJ. Activation of human umbilical vein endothelial cells leads to relocation and release of high-mobility group box chromosomal protein 1. Scandinavian Journal of Immunology. 2004;**60**:566–573.

Chapter 10

Bioactive Component of Licorice as an Antileishmanial Agent

Purnima Gupta , Anindita Ukil and Pijush K. Das

Additional information is available at the end of the chapter

http://dx.doi.org/10.5772/66289

Abstract

The term leishmaniasis encompasses a spectrum of vector-borne protozoan parasitic diseases ranging from self-healing cutaneous to fatal visceral leishmaniasis. The disease affects 12 million people worldwide with 0.5 million new cases per annum. Present antileishmanial chemotherapeutic drugs project limitations because of severe toxicity, lengthy regime and occurrence of resistance, thereby making development of newer, gentler and efficacious therapeutics an urgent need for treatment of leishmaniasis. Application of medicinal plants in treatment of refractory diseases is valued for its clinical efficacy and nontoxicity. The biologically active components derived from them continue to play important roles as chemopreventive agents. Licorice has been known for its medicinal property from ancient times for treatment of various ailments. 18β-Glycyrrhetinic acid, glycyrrhizic acid and licochalcone A are the most extensively studied constituents of licorice in terms of antileishmanial agent. Overall, this chapter is dedicated to highlight the current understanding of the mechanism of these bioactive constituents of licorice, which potentiates them as antileishmanial agents. Furthermore, it also brings to light the importance of folk medicine in curing diseases and thereby gives impetus to explore ancient medicines and thier mode of actions to use them progressively to cure diseases.

Keywords: 18β-glycyrrhetinic acid, glycyrrhizic acid, licochalcone A, antileishmanial, cytokines

1. Introduction

This chapter is dedicated to understand the mode of action of specific constituents of licorice, which have been isolated and characterized as antileishmanial agents. Among over 20 triterpinoids and 300 flavanoids present and characterized in licorice, only three, namely 18β-glycyrrhetinic acid, glycyrrhizin and licochalcone A, have been extensively studied for their antileishmanial properties. The structures of the compounds are given in **Figure 1**.

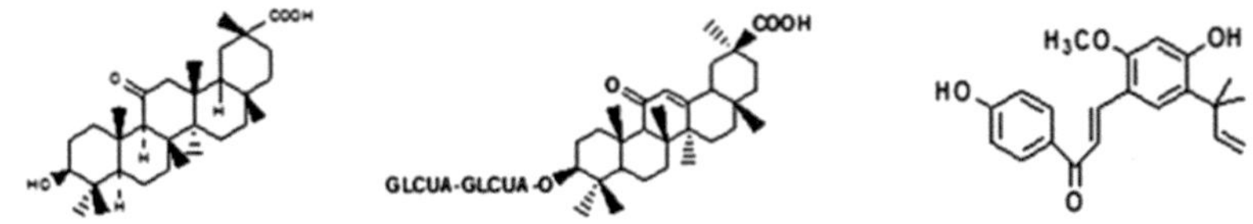

18β-Glycyrrhetinic Acid (GRA) Glycyrrhizin (GA) Licochalcone A (LCA)

Figure 1. Structure of the characterized antileishmanial constituents of licorice [1].

1.1. Leishmaniasis

Before going into the mechanistic details of these compounds, a brief idea about leishmaniasis will help understand the infection biology and the target of action of these molecules. *Leishmania* is a protozoan parasite that causes a spectrum of diseases ranging from the self-healing cutaneous to fatal visceral leishmaniasis. The visceral leishmaniasis particularly affects the spleen, liver and bone marrow [2]. It is highly endemic in the Indian subcontinent and East Africa. It is second only to malaria in annual worldwide fatalities due to protozoal infections [3–4].

1.2. Life cycle

Leishmania parasites remain in nature by transmission between the mammalian hosts through infected female sandfly bite. *Leishmania* lifecycle is characterized by having three developmental stages: procyclic promastigotes, metacyclic promastigotes and the amastigotes (**Figure 2**).

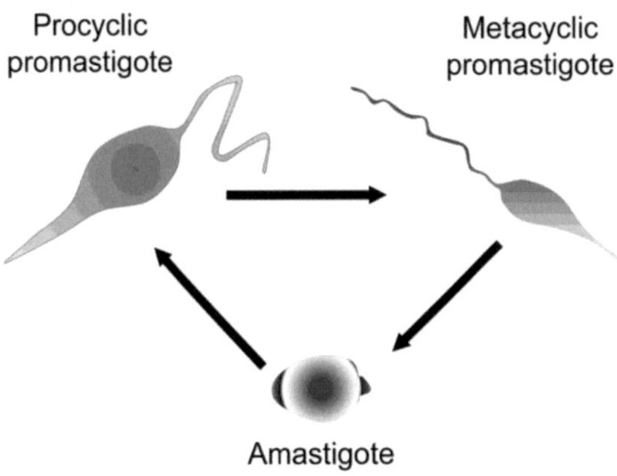

Figure 2. Lifecycle stages of *Leishmania sp* [2].

1.3. Transmission

In the sandfly (*Phlebotomus* and *Lutzomyia* spp) gut, the promastigote form of the parasite is seen which subsequently transforms to the infective metacyclic form which are regurgitated and injected in the skin of the mammalian host. Infected promastigotes then transforms to the amastigote form in the mammalian host. In a subsequent blood meal of this infected host, the amastigote forms are taken up which then transforms to the promastigotes in the gut and the cycle continues (**Figure 3**).

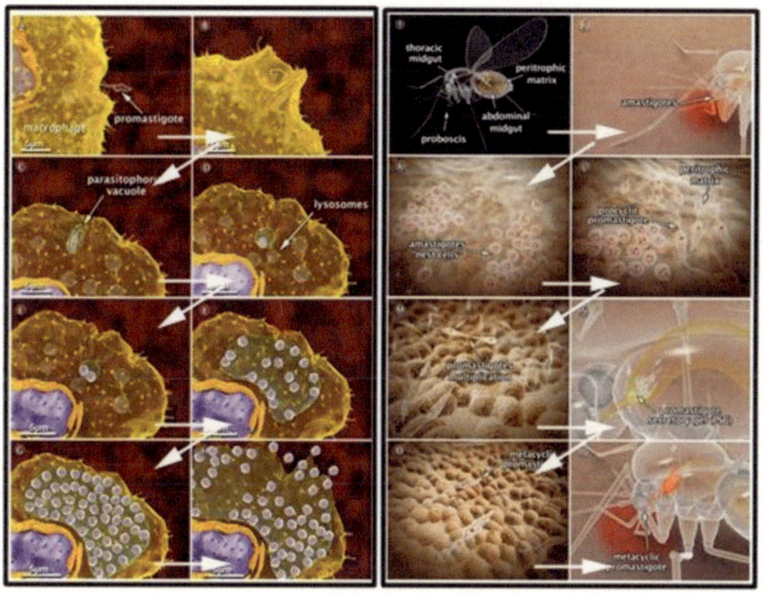

Figure 3. Schematic 3D view of the phases of interaction between the *Leishmania* parasite and sandfly and between the parasite and the vertebrate cells. "(A) Attachment of a promastigote to the macrophage surface. (B) The process of internalization via phagocytosis begins with the formation of pseudopods. (C) Leading to the formation of the parasitophorous vacuole (PV). In the PV, the promastigote transforms into an amastigote. (D) Recruitment and fusion of host cell lysosomes with the PV takes place. (E) In the PV, amastigotes divide several times. (F–G) Intense multiplication generates several hundreds of amastigotes. (H) The host cell bursts, and the parasites reach the extracellular space. (I) Schematic view of female sandfly showing the digestive tract. (J) During a blood meal, a female sandfly ingests infected macrophages with amastigote forms present in the blood of the vertebrate host. (K) Amastigotes form 'nest cells' in the abdominal midgut. (L) Amastigotes transform into procyclic promastigotes. (M) Promastigotes multiply and attach to the midgutepithelium. (N) Parasites migrate toward the anterior midgut, resume replication and start to produce promastigote secretory gel (PSG). (O) Promastigotes transform into infective metacyclic promastigotes. (P) Metacyclic promastigotes infect a new mammalian host via regurgitation during the blood meal. These images are based on micrographs obtained by scanning and transmission electron microscopy and by video microscopy" [5].

1.4. Disease manifestation

Visceral leishmaniasis patients show signs of systemic infection which include fever, fatigue, weakness, loss of appetite and weight loss. The parasite invades the blood and reticuloendothelial system, such as enlarged lymph nodes, spleen and liver. Darkening of the skin, popularly known as kala azar, which means black fever in Hindi, is infrequent. Anemia which is worsened by hypersplenism, leucopenia or thrombocytopenia, and hypergammaglobulinemia are characteristic. Untreated disease in any age group in time can produce profound cachexia, multisystem disease, bleeding, susceptibility to secondary infections and death [6].

1.5. Current treatment options

For visceral leishmaniasis, treatment is always recommended due to the fatal nature of the disease. The only treatment currently available for leishmaniasis relies on chemotherapy [7] as no vaccine has been successfully developed till date for humans. The first line of classical drug for treatment of leishmaniasis includes pentavalent antimonials, stibogluconate or meglumine antimonite. Pentavalent antimonials have been the drug of choice for more than 50 years [8–10]. Other common drugs are pentamidine, allopurinol, amphotericin B, imidazoles, miltefosine and paromomycin among others. Even though these drugs are effective other problems associated with these are (1) there lengthy regimens (weeks to months), (2) invasive modes of administration (intramuscular or intravenous) and (3) high drug-related toxicity along with the high cost of therapy which is beyond the capacity of many as this disease is known to be the 'disease of the poor'[10, 11]. All these factors together may lead to the patients discontinuing there therapies in the mid which have resulted in emergence of drug-resistant parasite strains adding to the list of problems associated with antileishmanial therapies [9, 11, 12].

To add to these overwhelming situations, emergence of coinfection collaterally with increasing incidences of HIV has decreased the number of options available to patients. As we will see in this chapter that immunosuppression is a key for parasite survival drugs, which can modulate host immune defenses, should be considered for effective treatment of leishmaniasis. Development of vaccines has remained a challenge; however, a canine vaccine has been developed, and it is in use in South America [13]. At present, no immunization options are available against leishmaniasis in humans.

1.6. Subversion of host defense

Like any other successful pathogens, *Leishmania* has also developed strategies to evade host immune mechanisms in order to survive within the host. A significant number of virulence factors discovered in *Leishmania* are directed against circumventing the host immune response. Apart from these, the parasite also has the ability to maintain a chronic infectious state within its host by modulation of regulatory factors, which exemplifies the extent on its immune evasion potential. Indeed, the ongoing battle between the robust immune response mounted by a host and the counter evasion strategies by the parasite ultimately decides the fate of the disease.

All these further establishes the fact that a chemotherapeutic alone is not enough to treat this intelligent parasite, and indeed an immunomodulator which can activate hosts own defense mechanism will be a better adjunct to the current line of treatment, which is relatively better in terms of toxicity, efficacy and mode of administration.

http://dx.doi.org/10.5772/66289

2. 18β-Glycyrrhetinic acid (GRA)

18β-Glycyrrhetinic acid (GRA), a pentacyclic triterpene derivative of the β-amyrin type, is obtained from the roots of *Glycyrrhizza glabra* L. It is known to exhibit a variety of pharmacological effects like antiulcerative, anti-hepatotoxic, anti-tumorigenic and immunoregulatory activities [14–17]. As evident, GRA has potent immunomodulatory effects, thus its potency as an antileishmanial agent and the underlying mechanism was thoroughly explored.

2.1. Cytotoxicity

The first and foremost criteria for evaluation of a drug for its antiparasitic activity would be to evaluate its cytotoxic effects. The development of new drugs that has immunomodulatory properties requires both pharmacokinetic and toxicity studies to be carried out in conjunction to clinical verification. Our work so far has shown that GRA is relatively a nontoxic compound with up to 1.5 g/day consumption in humans [18].

GRA exhibited potent in vitro activity against intracellular *L. donovani* amastigotes (IC_{50}, 4.3 μg/ml); it was devoid of any obvious cytotoxicity on macrophage host cells, because the cytotoxic concentration causing 50% cell death was ~100 μg/ml [19]. The infected mice treated with GRA were completely cured. Moreover, this therapy was seen to be effective in mice with established disease-progressive Th2 response. After treatment and resolution of parasitism, the cytokine profile indicated a switch to a protective Th1 pattern associated with upregulation of NO [19].

2.2. Mechanism

2.2.1. Macrophage activation by NF-κB-mediated nitric oxide and proinflammatory cytokine production

Once the cytotoxic parameters were found satisfying the mechanistic profile was explored. The disease resolving property of GRA could be attributed to the production of NO and proinflammatory cytokines such as IL-12 [20, 21]. The most diversely studied mechanism that assists the *Leishmania* survival is modulating the macrophage cytokines production to bias the immune response to its benefit [22, 23]. *Leishmania* mainly inhibits the secretion of macrophage proinflammatory or disease resolving cytokines, which include interleukin 12 (IL-12), tumor necrosis factor alpha (TNF-α), interferon gamma (IFN-γ) and aids the secretion of anti-inflammatory or disease promoting cytokines interleukin 10 (IL-10), transforming growth factor beta (TGF-β) for its own benefit.

Cytokine IL-12 is downregulated by *Leishmania via* ligation with macrophage receptors [22, 23]. One of the most important initial signaling events is the release of IL-12 by the infected macrophage, leading to subsequent priming of the Th1 response and production of IFN-γ [5, 24–26]. *Leishmania* also upregulates the production of anti-inflammatory cytokines such as IL-10. IL-10 is important in suppressing macrophage leishmanicidal activity by opposing IFN-γ [22, 24, 27], nitric oxide (NO) and IL-12 production [28].

The killing of intracellular *Leishmania* parasites by GRA correlated with the induction of the iNOS pathway. Nitric oxide (NO) is known to mediate many of the cytotoxic and immunological effects upon pathogenic challenge. This NO production has been shown to be dependent upon the inducible for of the nitric oxide synthases (iNOS) [29], whereas under normal physiological conditions only the constituitive forms of NOS (cNOS) are functional. Induction of iNOS in turn is under transcriptional regulation of NF-κB, a group of transcription factors that belong to the Rel protein family. The activated form of NF-κB is a heterodimer, which usually consists of two proteins, p65 (RelA) and p50 subunit [30]. In unstimulated cells, NF-κB is found in the cytoplasm bound to an inhibitor, inhibitor of nuclear factor κB (IκB)α and IκBβ [31]. This association prevents nuclear translocation of NF-κB and hence iNOS transcription and NO production. Upon pathogenic challenge, the large multisubunit protein kinase, inhibitor of nuclear factor kappa-B kinase subunit beta(IKK) causes rapid proteasomal degradation of IκBα, thereby releasing NFκB and allowing its nuclear translocation. This event is inhibited in *Leishmania donovani* infection thereby promoting parasite survival [19] (**Figure 4**).

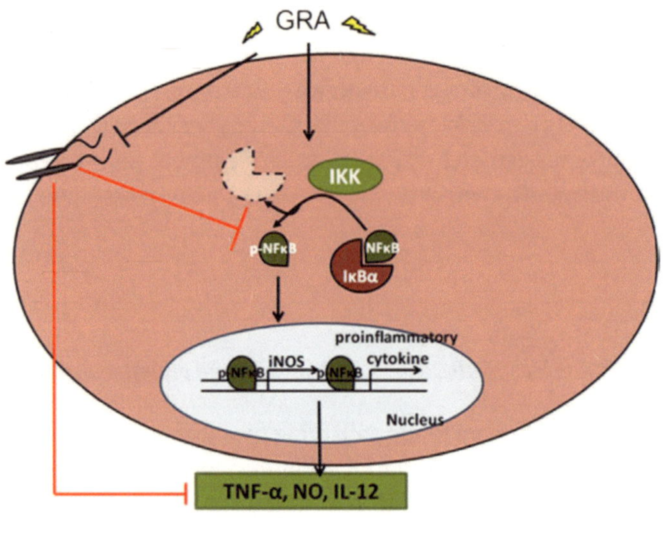

Figure 4. GRA promotes NF-κB-mediated parasite killing.

GRA, on the other hand, activates NF-κB through the regulation of genes essentially involved in encoding proinflammatory cytokines and inflammatory mediators such as NO. *L. donovani* infection suppressed NF-κB activation and translocation which was restored upon GRA administration via induction of IκBα phosphorylation. This in turn was achieved by modulating the upstream signal leading to IKK (inhibitor of nuclear factor kappa-B kinase subunit beta) activation, that is, without directly interfering with IKK (inhibitor of nuclear factor kappa-B kinase subunit beta). Overall this signaling activation by GRA led to degradation of IκBα leading to the translocation of NF-κB in the nucleus and transcriptional activation of iNOS and proinflammatory cytokines [19] (**Figure 4**). The antileishmanial activity of GRA was dependent on the iNOS activity and NO production was further justified by addition of a specific NOS inhibitor, N^G-monomethyl-L-arginine (NMMA). Upon administration of NMMA along with GRA, a reduction in the parasite killing capability of GRA was seen and withdrawal of NMMA led to decreased parasite survival indicating a role of GRA-induced NO-mediated parasite killing.

2.2.2. *MAPK and phosphatases*

Mitogen-activated protein kinase(MAPK) plays an important role in activation of NF-κB. MAPK signaling cascades are rather complex events which ultimately results in manifold increase in stimulus-mediated responses. However, if this response remains unchecked, it may be detrimental for the cells and thus a balance between the activity of the kinases and phosphatases play important roles in physiological scenario. In macrophages, the MAPK (mitogen-activated protein kinase) cascade and the NF-κB pathway play important roles in the regulation of functions involved in inflammation and host defense. *L. donovani* successfully sabotage these pathways creating an anti-inflammatory milieu by inhibiting production of NO and proinflammatory cytokines thereby strengthening their existence within the macrophages [32]. Thus, the agents that can activate NF-κB pathway creating a proinflammtory milieu potent enough to kill the parasites might prove attractive candidates to control *Leishmania* infection. Our studies also revealed that the Mitogen-activated protein kinase kinase - extracellular signal regulated kinases (MEK-ERK) pathway is compensated in infected cells [33]. GRA, the triterpenoid is an ideal candidate both because of its pharmacologically safe parameters and immunomodulatory properties [19]. The switching of the immunological response was found to be dependent upon the MAPK (mitogen-activated protein kinase) activation among which

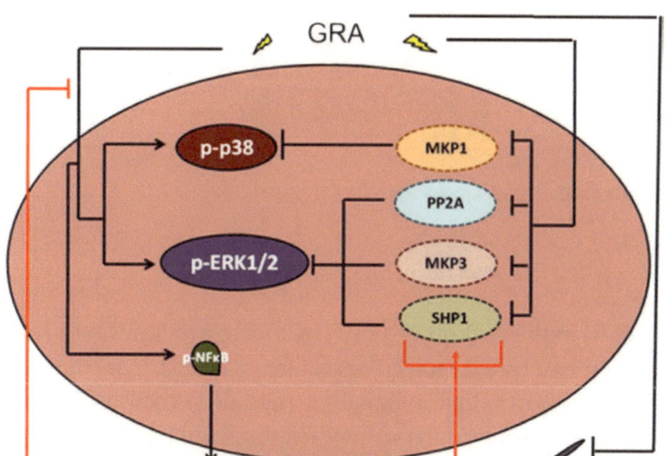

Figure 5. The balance between kinases and phosphatases is restored upon GRA treatment.

only ERK and p38 were found to be regulated by GRA [34]. In *Leishmania* infection, these MAPK (mitogen-activated protein kinase) activation was severely compensated which was in turn is attributed to the fact that activity of MAPK (mitogen-activated protein kinase) phosphatases, which dephosphorylate and thereby inactivate MAPK (mitogen-activated protein kinase), significantly increased. This corroborated with the fact that inhibition of SHP-1, a MAPK (mitogen-activated protein kinase) phosphatase led to stronger proinflammatory responses against infection [35]. However, GRA treatment could potentially inhibit the activity of the phosphatases, thereby shifting the total kinase to phosphatase balance in favor of creating an antileishmanial milieu [34] (**Figure 5**).

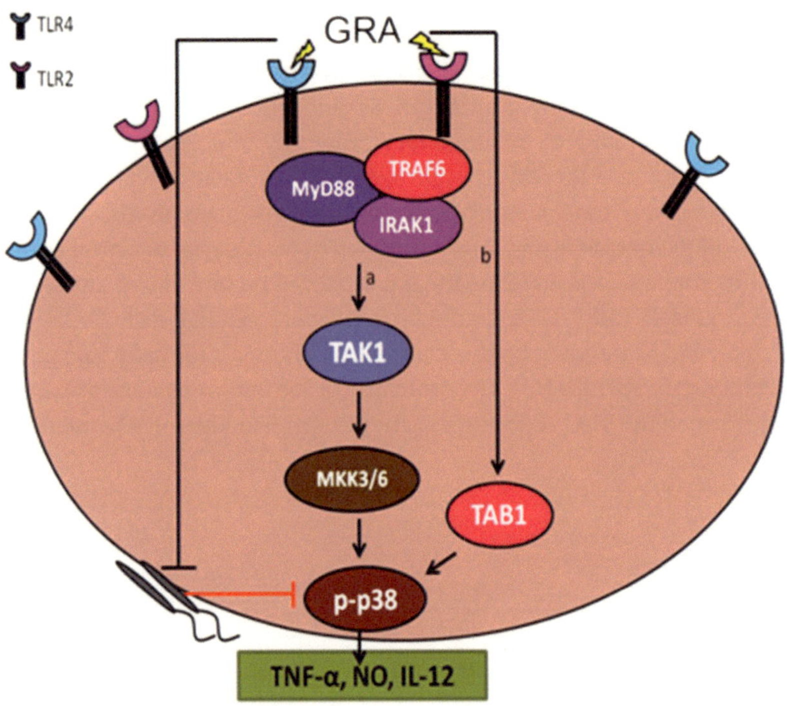

Figure 6. GRA activates p38 via the TLR2/4 pathway.

2.2.3. Downregulation of toll-like receptor (TLR) pathways

Toll-like receptor (TLR) expressed on the cells of the innate immune system are critical for recognition of pathogen-associated molecular patterns (PAMP). Upon ligand binding, the TLR gets activated leading to downstream signaling cascade activation leading to NF-κB- and MAPK (mitogen-activated protein kinase)-mediated proinflammatory cytokine production. The TLR2 agonists used to activate TLR2 signaling pathway showed host protective immune response resulting in parasite clearance from *L. donovani* infected macrophages [36]. To subvert this inflammatory response *Leishmania* either recruits suppressors of the cytokine signaling (SOCS) family proteins, SOCS-1/3 [37], or activates host de-ubiquitinating enzyme A20 to negatively regulate TLR2/4-induced host protective response [38, 39]. *Leishmania* can alter TLR4 signaling to favor its establishment within the macrophages. TLR4-mediated macrophage activation was shown to be suppressed in *Leishmania* infection through the release of TGF-β [40]. *L. mexicana* capitalizes on TLR4 signaling to inhibit the production of IL-12 by infected macrophages and promotes parasite establishment [41]. Other TLRs involved in infection with *Leishmania* include TLR3 and TLR9.

The effect of GRA is mediated by means of MAPK (mitogen-activated protein kinase) activation and phosphatase downregulation. Deeper analysis revealed that the MAPK (mitogen-activated protein kinase) p38 activation was dependent on GRA-mediated canonical and noncanonical activation where numerous upstream molecules play important roles [42]. This study further highlighted the importance of p38 MAPK (mitogen-activated protein kinase) in GRA-mediated parasite elimination and its activation by upstream kinases like MKK3/6 which itself is dependent upon upstream signaling molecules (**Figure 6**).

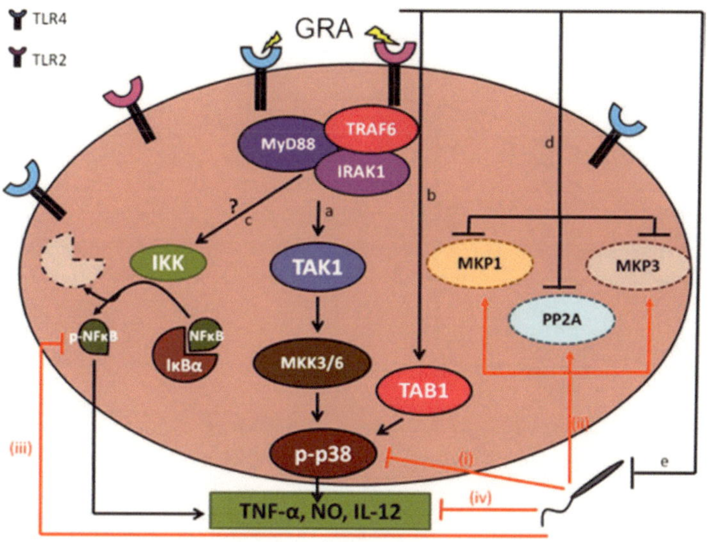

Figure 7. Mode of Action of 18β-Glycyrrhetinic Acid-potent antileishmanial immunomodulator. *Leishmania* (i) inhibits p38 phosphorylation, (ii) activates phosphatases, (iii) inhibit activation of NFκB thereby leading to (iv) inhibition of proinflammatory cytokine reponses. 18β-Glycyrrhetinic Acid acts as an immunomodulator which in infection activates (a) canonical and (b) non canonical pathways leading to phosphorylation and activation of p38, (c) activates IκB Kinase which in turn results in IκBα phosphorylation and degradation leading to NFκB phosphorylation and activation, (d) inhibit phosphatases which would otherwise lead to dephosphorylation and inhibition of major kinases therby promoting proinflammatory cytokine response generation and (e) parasite killing.

Thus, the effective macrophage activation via NO and proinflammatory cytokines production in response to GRA treatment justifies the candidature of this potent immunomodulator as an antileishmanial. Furthermore, this compound may prove to be effective in terms of generating immunity not only in nonhealing leishmaniasis but also for the treatment of other chronic infectious diseases. A comprehensive model giving the overall mechanistic insight into the mode of action of GRA as antileishmanial agent will help in deducing its function in other intramacrophage pathogens which assume similar immunoevasive mechanisms to escape host defenses (**Figure 7**).

3. Glycyrrhizic acid

Another constituent of licorice, which serves as an antileishmanial compound, is glycyrrhizic acid (GA) [43]. The studies using this compound showed an increase in NO production with restoration of Th1 cytokine balance and inhibition of immunosuppressive prostaglandin E2(PGE2) production. This is in line with recent evidences, which suggests that the parasite is able to induce PGE2 production via promoting inducible COX2 expression. This in turn resulted in activation of EP receptors (PGE2 receptors) on the host cell surface thereby causing Cyclic adenosine monophosphate(cAMP) induction and cytokine production [44] (**Figure 8**).

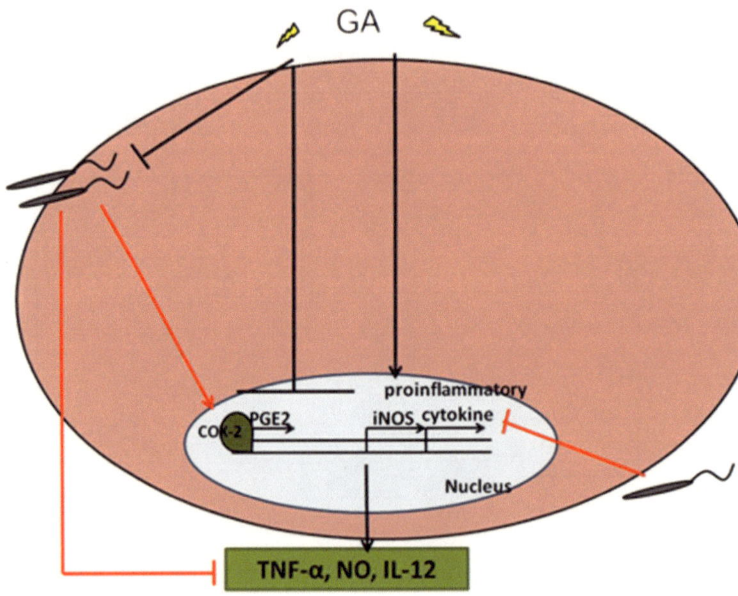

Figure 8. Glycyrrhizic acid mediated PGE2 inhibition and NO and proinflammatory cytokine production helps parasite suppression.

This is also anticipated as glycyrrhizic acid is readily hydrolyzed to glycyrrhetinic acid in human body [45] which is already discussed in details to have antileishmanial activities. Recent studies further shows that this compound when used in conjunction with antimonials can help in overcoming the resistance seen in the antimony resistant parasites. Extensive use of the antimonials and low follow-up of cases had led to emergence of antimonial resistant strains of the parasite [46]. The main criteria for this resistance is attributed to the overexpression and

http://dx.doi.org/10.5772/66289

efflux activity of a class of transporters on the surface of the host cells namely P-glycoprotein (P-gp) and multidrug resistance-associated protein (MRP-1) thereby leading to efflux of the antimonials and parasite persistence. However, administration of glycyrrhizin led to suppression of these transporters and simultaneously shifted the overall anti-inflammatory milieu to the proinflammatory one [46] (**Figure 9**). Thus, this herbal compound can serve as an economical effective counterpart to its expensive counterparts like miltefosine and amphotericin B.

Further studies demonstrated the role of glycyrrhizin in mediating proliferation of T cells, thereby promoting disease resolving IFN-γ production in *Leishmania* infected cells. This was in turn an effect of suppression of COX-2 by glycyrrhizin on the myeloid-derived suppressor cells, a heterogeneous population of precursor cells, which promotes parasite survival by suppressing T cell functions [47].

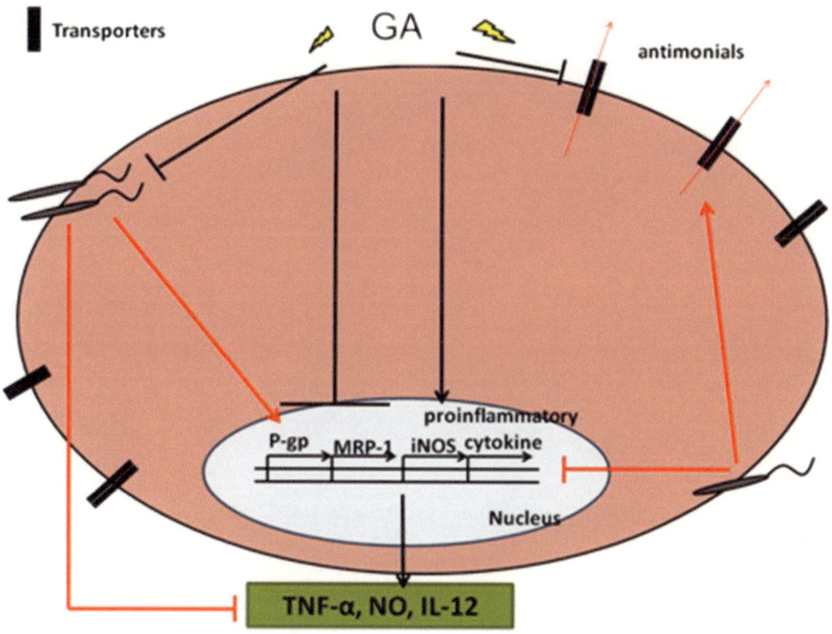

Figure 9. Glycyyrhizic acid (GA) suppresses P-gp and MRP-1 activation leading to antimonial retention and parasite inhibition.

4. Licochalcone A

The oxygenated chalcone, licochalcone A, has also been extensively studied to understand the mechanism of this compound as an antileishmanial agent [48–50]. Previous studies have shown its effect as antioxidant, antimicrobial and anti-tumor promoting properties [51, 52]. The use of this compound in infection particularly affected the amastigote forms of the parasite and to a lesser extent the promastigote form having practically no effect on the host monocytes even at higher concentrations. The main target of licochalcone A was the mitochondrion of the parasite, whereas the host mitochondrion remained unaffected [48]. The reason for the same is still unknown but further studies suggested that the parasite respiratory rate was affected resulting in an overall decrease in parasite O_2 consumption and CO_2 production with a decrease in the activity of the mitochondrial dehydrogenases [50]. In vivo studies also showed high parasite elimination in in vivo studies upon intraperitoneal administration of licochalcone A as opposed to intralesional or oral administration [49]. All these findings suggests potential role of licochalcone A as an antileishmanial agent although studies understanding the mechanism of this compound is still underway (**Figure 10**).

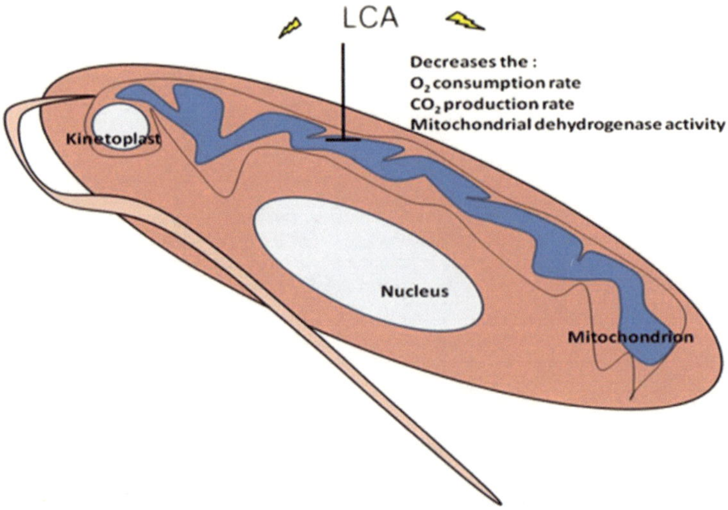

Figure 10. The effect of licochalcone A on the mitochondrion of the *Leishmania* parasite.

5. Conclusion

All these compounds have effectively showed their potential as antileishmanial agents. Future works leading to clinical trials of these compounds alone or in conjunction with present chemotherapeutics may highly benefit the *Leishmania* distressed people. Overall the immunomodulators of the herbal origin like licorice and its constituents open up avenues for formulation of cost-effective and low-toxicity drugs for diseases with limited treatment.

Acknowledgements

We would like to acknowledge all our funding agencies, past and present: University Grants Commission, Council of Scientific & Industrial Research (CSIR), National Academy of

Sciences, India (NASI), Department of Science and Technology, Department of Biotechnology (DBT), Government of West Bengal, Department of Biotechnology and our university and institute: University of Calcutta and Indian Institute of Chemical Biology.

Author details

Purnima Gupta[1], Anindita Ukil[1] and Pijush K. Das[2*]

*Address all correspondence to: pijushdas@iicb.res.in

1 Department of Biochemistry, University of Calcutta, Kolkata, India

2 Infectious Diseases and Immunology Division, Indian Institute of Chemical Biology, Kolkata, India

References

[1] Wang L, Yang R, et al. 2015. The antiviral and antimicrobial activities of licorice, a widely-used Chinese herb. Acta pharmaceutica sinica B. 5:310–5.

[2] Neva FA, Brown HW. 1994. Basic clinical parasitology. Appleton & Lange, U.S.

[3] Barbieri CL. 2006. Immunology of canine leishmaniasis. Parasite immunology 28: 329–37.

[4] Solano-Gallego L, Koutinas A, et al. 2009. Directions for the diagnosis, clinical staging, treatment and prevention of canine leishmaniosis. Veterinary parasitology 165: 1–18.

[5] Teixeira DE, Benchimol M, Rodrigues JC, Crepaldi PH, Pimenta PF, de Souza W. 2013. The cell biology of *Leishmania*: how to teach using animations. PLoS pathogens 9: e1003594.

[6] Davidson RN. 1998. Practical guide for the treatment of leishmaniasis. Drugs 56: 1009–18.

[7] Davis AJ, Murray HW, Handman E. 2004. Drugs against leishmaniasis: a synergy of technology and partnerships. Trends in parasitology 20: 73–6.

[8] Frezard F, Demicheli C, Ribeiro RR. 2009. Pentavalent antimonials: new perspectives for old drugs. Molecules 14: 2317–36.

[9] Herwaldt BL. 1999. Leishmaniasis. Lancet 354: 1191–9.

[10] Reithinger R, Dujardin JC, Louzir H, Pirmez C, Alexander B, Brooker S. 2007. Cutaneous leishmaniasis. The Lancet. Infectious diseases 7: 581–96.

[11] Chappuis F, Sundar S, et al. 2007. Visceral leishmaniasis: what are the needs for diagnosis, treatment and control? Nature reviews microbiology 5: 873–82.

[12] Bailey MS, Lockwood DN. 2007. Cutaneous leishmaniasis. Clinics in dermatology 25: 203–11.

[13] Dantas-Torres F. 2006. Leishmune vaccine: the newest tool for prevention and control of canine visceral leishmaniosis and its potential as a transmission-blocking vaccine. Veterinary parasitology 141: 1–8.

[14] Rossi T, Galatulas I, et al. 1995. Influence of glycyrrhizin on the evolution and respiration of Ehrlich ascites tumour cells. In vivo 9: 183–6.

[15] Kroes BH, Beukelman CJ, et al. 1997. Inhibition of human complement by beta-glycyrrhetinic acid. Immunology 90: 115–20.

[16] Farina C, Pinza M, et al. 1998. Synthesis and anti-ulcer activity of new derivatives of glycyrrhetic, oleanolic and ursolic acids. Farmaco 53: 22–32.

[17] Jeong HG, You HJ, et al. 2002. Hepatoprotective effects of 18beta-glycyrrhetinic acid on carbon tetrachloride-induced liver injury: inhibition of cytochrome P450 2E1 expression. Pharmacological research 46: 221–27.

[18] Krahenbuhl S, Hasler F, et al. 1994. Kinetics and dynamics of orally administered 18β-glycyrrhetinic acid in humans. Journal of clinical endocrinology & metabolism. 78: 581–5.

[19] Ukil A, Biswas A, et al. 2005. 18β-glycyrrhetinic acid triggers curative Th1 response and nitric oxide up-regulation in experimental visceral leishmaniasis associated with the activation of NF-kappa B. Journal of immunology 175: 1161–9.

[20] Jeong HG, Kim JY. 2002. Induction of inducible nitric oxide synthase expression by 18-β-glycyrrhetinic acid in macrophages. FEBS letter 523: 208–12.

[21] Dai JH, Iwatani Y., et al. 2001. Glycyrrhizin enhances interleukin-12 production in peritoneal macrophages. Immunology 103: 235–43.

[22] Cunningham AC. 2002. Parasitic adaptive mechanisms in infection by *Leishmania*. Experimental and molecular pathology 72: 132–41.

[23] Kane MM, Mosser DM. 2000. *Leishmania* parasites and their ploys to disrupt macrophage activation. Current opinion in hematology 7: 26–31.

[24] Barral-Netto M, Brodskyn C, Carvalho EM, Barral A. 1998. Human_leishmaniasis/cytokines.bahia.br. Brazilian journal of medical and biological research = Revista brasileira de pesquisas medicas e biologicas/Sociedade Brasileira de Biofisica ... [et al.] 31: 149–55.

[25] Piedrafita D, Proudfoot L, et al. 1999. Regulation of macrophage IL-12 synthesis by *Leishmania* phosphoglycans. European journal of immunology 29: 235–44.

[26] Reiner SL, Locksley RM. 1995. The regulation of immunity to *Leishmania major*. Annual review of immunology 13: 151–77.

[27] Belkaid Y, Hoffmann KF, et al. 2001. The role of interleukin (IL)-10 in the persistence of *Leishmania major* in the skin after healing and the therapeutic potential of anti-IL-10 receptor antibody for sterile cure. The journal of experimental medicine 194: 1497–506.

[28] Olivier M, Gregory DJ, Forget G. 2005. Subversion mechanisms by which *Leishmania* parasites can escape the host immune response: a signaling point of view. Clinical microbiology reviews 18: 293–305.

[29] Manna PP, Bharadwaj D, et al. 1993. Impairment of natural killer cell activity in Indian Kala-azar: restoration of activity by interleukin 2 but not by α or γ interferon. Infection and immunity 61: 3565–9.

[30] Baldwin AS. 1996. The NF-κB and IκB proteins: new discoveries and insights. Annual review immunology 14: 649–83.

[31] May MJ, Ghosh S. 1998. Signal transduction through NF-κB. Immunology today 19: 80–8.

[32] Prive C, Descoteaux A. 2000. *Leishmania donovani* promastigotes evade the activation of mitogen-activated protein kinases p38, c-Jun N-terminal kinase and extracellular signal-regulated kinase-1/2 during infection of naı¨ve macrophages. European journal of immunology 8: 2235–44.

[33] Kar S, Ukil A, et al. 2011. Cystatin cures visceral leishmaniasis by NF-κB-mediated proinflammatory response through co-ordination of TLR/MyD88 signaling with p105-Tpl2-ERK pathway. European journal of immunology 41: 116–27.

[34] Ukil A., Kar S, et al. 2011. Curative effect of 18beta-glycyrrhetinic acid in experimental visceral leishmaniasis depends on phosphatase-dependent modulation of cellular MAP kinases. PLoS one 6: e29062.

[35] Forget G, Matte C, et al. 2005. Regulation of the *Leishmania*-induced innate inflammatory response by the protein tyrosine phosphatase SHP-1. European journal of immunology 35: 1906–17.

[36] Bhattacharya P, Bhattacharjee S, et al. 2010. Arabinosylated lipoarabinomannan-mediated protection in visceral leishmaniasis through up-regulation of toll-like receptor 2 signaling: an immunoprophylactic approach. The journal of infectious diseases 202: 145–55.

[37] de Veer MJ, Curtis JM, et al. 2003. MyD88 is essential for clearance of *Leishmania major:* possible role for lipophosphoglycan and Toll-like receptor 2 signaling. European journal of immunology 33: 2822–31.

[38] Srivastav S, Kar S, Chande AG, Mukhopadhyaya R, Das PK. 2012. *Leishmania donovani* exploits host deubiquitinating enzyme A20, a negative regulator of TLR signaling, to subvert host immune response. Journal of immunology 189: 924–34.

[39] Gupta P, Giri J, et al. 2014. *Leishmania donovani* targets tumor necrosis factor receptor-associated factor (TRAF) 3 for impairing TLR4-mediated host response. FASEB journal: official publication of the Federation of American Societies for Experimental Biology 28: 1756–68.

[40] Das S, Pandey K, et al. 2012. TGF-beta1 re-programs TLR4 signaling in L. donovani infection: enhancement of SHP-1 and ubiquitin-editing enzyme A20. Immunology and cell biology 90: 640–54.

[41] Shweash M, Adrienne McGachy H, et al. 2011. *Leishmania mexicana* promastigotes inhibit macrophage IL-12 production via TLR-4 dependent COX-2, iNOS and arginase-1 expression. Molecular immunology 48: 1800–8.

[42] Gupta P, Ukil A, et al. 2015. Antileishmanial effect of 18β-glycyrrhetinic acid is mediated by Toll-like receptor-dependent canonical and noncanonical p38 activation. Antimicrobial agents and chemotherapy 59: 2531–9.

[43] Bhattacharjee S, Bhattacharjee A, et al. 2012. Glycyrrhizic acid suppresses Cox-2-mediated anti-inflammatory responses during *Leishmania donovani* infection. Journal of antimicrobial chemotherapy 67: 1905–14.

[44] Saha A, Biswas A, et al. 2014. Prostaglandin E2 negatively regulates the production of inflammatory cytokines/chemokines and IL-17 in visceral leishmaniasis. Journal of immunology 193: 2330–9.

[45] Huang RY, Chu YL, et al. 2014. 18β-Glycyrrhetinic acid suppresses cell proliferation through inhibiting thromboxane synthase in non-small cell lung cancer. PLoS one 9: e93690.

[46] Bhattacharjee A, Majumder S, et al. 2015. Co-administration of glycyrrhizic acid with the antileishmanial drug sodium antimony gluconate (SAG) cures SAG-resistant visceral leishmaniasis. International journal of antimicrobial agents 45: 268–77.

[47] Bandyopadhyay S, Bhattacharjee A, et al. 2015. Glycyrrhizic acid-mediated subdual of myeloid-derived suppressor cells induces antileishmanial immune responses in a susceptible host. Infection and immunity. 83: 4476–86.

[48] Chen M, Christensen SB, et al. 1993. Licochalcone A, a novel antiparasitic agent with potent activity against human pathogenic protozoan species of *Leishmania*. Antimicrobial agents and chemotherapy 37: 2550–6.

[49] Chen M, Christensen SB, et al. 1994. Antileishmanial activity of licochalcone A in mice infected with *Leishmania major* and in hamsters infected with *Leishmania donovani*. Antimicrobial agents and chemotherapy 38: 1339–44.

[50] Zhai L, Blom J, et al. 1995. The antileishmanial agent licochalcone A interferes with the function of parasite mitochondria. Antimicrobial agents and chemotherapy 39: 2742–8.

[51] Okada K, Tamura Y, et al. 1989. Identification of antimicrobial and antioxidant constituents from licorice of Russian and Xinjiang origin. Chemical & pharmaceutical bulletin 37: 2528–30.

[52] Shibata S, Inoue H., et al. 1991. Inhibitory effects of licochalcone A isolated from *Glycyrrhiza inflata* root on inflammatory ear edema and tumour promotion in mice. Planta medica 57: 221–4.